Foundation of Physical Education

Foundation of Physical Education

Edited & Compiled by

Dr. H. Sharadrao
B.Sc., M.P.E., Ph.D., NIS, D.Ye.
Director (Physical Education)
Government of Maharashtra's Rajaram College
Kolhapur (Maharashtra)

SPORTS PUBLICATION
7/26, Ground Floor, Ansari Road,
Darya Ganj, New Delhi-110002
Phones: (Office) 65749511 (Fax) 011-23240261
(Mobile) 9868028838 (Residence) 27562163
E-mail: lakshaythani@hotmail.com

Published by:

SPORTS PUBLICATION
7/26, Ground Floor, Ansari Road, Darya Ganj, New Delhi-110002
Ph. : (Office) 65749511, 23240261 (Mobile) 9868028838
(Residence) 27562163 (Fax) 011-23240261
E-mail: *lakshaythani@hotmail.com*

I.S.B.N: 978-81-7879-551-5

PRINTED IN INDIA 2009

Laser Typeset by:
JAIN MEDIA GRAPHICS,
C-4/95-A, Keshav Puram, Delhi-35.

Printed by:
CHAWLA OFFSET PRINTERS, Delhi-110052

Price: Rs. 395/-

CONTENTS

1

EDUCATION—MEANING, AIMS AND OBJECTIVES

INTRODUCTION

Man is considered the most valuable and superior creature of God. One of an important ability which a man has and which makes him superior to other animals is his ability to learn. Human beings has got intelligence. It does not imply that all the other creatures of the world do not have intelligence. Animals also possess some degree of intelligence, but the intelligence which human beings have enable them to modify his animal tendencies as needed by the society. Man can adapt himself according to the environment in which he lives.

The intelligence of a human being can be enhanced with the help of education. Proper education can develop the capabilities of a human being and it also helps in acquiring a conductive attitude. Conductive attitude is very important for being a human being.

Various experts have defined the concept of education differently. For instance, Prof. Drever has defined it as a process with the help of which one can give a proper shape to the knowledge, character and behaviour of someone. In other words, education is a constructive process which can lead to enlightenment and can develop various aspects of an individual's personality.

With the help of proper education, there can be physical development, mental development and social development also. Another expert, P.C. Banerji has said that education helps in developing the power of adaptation to an ever changing social environment. Thus one thing Banerji has made clear is that nature and outlook of society keeps on changing, and society is being made by people living in it and outlook of society changes when the nature of behaviour of people living in it change. Kant has stated that education is an important development in an individual of all the perfections of which he is capable.

Thus, it can be said that education results in an integrated, balanced and all-round development of an individual, which can help him in becoming a civilised and responsible member of the society. Education provides a man dynamic personality which provide him maturity and help him in becoming a more maturer person.

From time to time, things keep on changing. It can be said that change is the law of nature. As the development take place in various areas, people feel needs of new things. For instance, fundamental needs or requirements of primitive man were food, shelter and clothing. With the progress of the society, today, man's needs have changed to a lot of extent. Into various biological, sociological and psychological aspects of life, one can easily categorise these new developed needs. Necessity is the mother of invention, because of which when man realized the need of new things, he also develop the means to get them fulfilled. Now the factor which is responsible for the development is nothing but the knowledge. The reason today's man is considered quite developed in comparison to primitive man is his knowledge. This knowledge is gained from the education.

It can be said that education helps in developing the overall personality of an individual. If it is said that education is an important tool to grow and develop the personality of an individually, it will not be wrong in any way. Education not only helps in developing an individual, but indirectly it also help in developing the society as society is made up of human beings and it is with the growth and development of people living in that society will develop and grow.

Some people consider education to be a mere transmission of one kind of knowledge into another, but it is not right or fair. It is not proper to analyse the value of education in terms of knowledge that gets transmitted, as the difference in the behaviour of person that education brings should be the real criterion. For this reason, education not only transmits one kind of knowledge into another, but it also affects the behaviour of persons getting it. An important test of the education is not only knowledge, but it is also performance or behaviour of the person that is being counted.

DIFFERENT ASPECTS OF EDUCATION

It is not an easy task to define the word education as it is very broad in nature. Education provides a precise meaning. Education has a very complicated nature as it deals with human beings and human beings have an ever progressive nature. Moreover, the society in which human beings live is also keeps on changing and in this kind of condition, it is really not easy to provide a proper definition of concept of Education.

According to the different life situations, definition

of concept of education keeps on changing. There are various theories dealing with the origin of concept of education. According to one theory, word education has been derived from a Latin word Educere which implies to lead out and to bring forth. On the basis of the word from where word education is being derived, some experts define it as a means to lead out a human being and to bring forth or develop the abilities he possess. Whatever one man possess inside him, i.e., knowledge, power, ability, it is with the help of education that can be bring out or can be developed.

According to another school of experts, the word education has been derived from a Latin word 'Education' which is formed of two distinct words, namely, 'e' and 'duco'. In literal sense, word 'e' implies out of and word 'duco' implies to lead out. When these two words combine with each other, the concept that emerges out is a process which helps in developing one's inner abilities or which brings out the inner capabilities of a human being.

According to T.P. Nunn, education helps in developing the individuality of a child with the help of which he can contribute human life in accordance with his utmost capabilities.

On the basis of above discussion, it can be said that knowledge exists nowhere but in the interior of a human being and to draw that interior knowledge is the main objective or function of education. For drawing out the interior knowledge, it is very necessary to use some kind of method or means. It can be said that in order to draw out interior abilities or knowledge, one has to put something it. To get the output, one has to use input. For this reason, it is necessary to provide knowledge, experience and information to a human being and after this only we can get or draw out of him the best abilities in him.

There lies some inner capacities, which are there in a human being right from the birth. This capability is termed as the innate capacity to learn. This capacity can also be developed with the help of education. It can be said that education is such a process which result in a progressive and systematic development of man's all inner abilities. Process of education is continuous in nature. In other words, it is a never ending process. It can be viewed as a progress and development which cannot be stopped. Throughout the life, one can easily see the importance and place of education in the life. Generations get change, but value of education remains the same.

Education provides one the ability to think creatively, it provide it reasoning power and analytical ability. These abilities helps an individual to act and adapt oneself in changing society. With the help of these abilities, one can very easily adapt oneself according to the social scenario. Education also brings a complete change or development in the personality of a man. Some experts have said that education is that process of living in which common reconstruction of experiences are included. It leads to development of those qualities in an individual which will help him in controlling the environment. It can said that education leads a kind of change or modifies one in such a way that individual can adapt himself in the changed conditions.

There are two views or aspects in seeing something, namely, the broader and narrow. In the same way, we can also view the education in broader as well as in narrow sense.

BROADER VIEW OF EDUCATION

We have broader meaning of education according to which it is such a long process which remains active throughout the life. In this kind of thinking, life is considered as a kind of school and the perfect age for learning is throughout the life. Life consists of various areas which affect ourselves in one way or other. If we interpret the meaning of education in broader sense, it is not limited merely to educational institutions but it is an indirect process as well as incidental. There is no specific time period in which process of education takes place, but it is throughout the lifetime of an individual in which this process takes place.

It can be said that education is such a process which begins from the birth of an individual and continues till the end of life. According to this thought of school, an individual learns throughout the life and there are various teachers in different forms. For instance, at home, he learns from his parents, his elders and even sometimes from his younger ones. In the school, he learns from his teachers and class mates. In office or life after school, he learns from officers and colleagues. Thus, this process of learning goes on and from various persons, individual keeps on learning something, however, the role of teacher is done by different persons from time to time.

Whatever the level of education, one cannot completely be called educated as process of education is never ending. The life pattern of every society keeps on changing from time to time and one has to change himself according to such changed pattern. These necessary changes which one has to bring in himself is brought to a lot of extent with the help of education.

Some people consider education only restricted to class-room, but this is a myth as education continues even outside the classroom in various ways. There is no age group or sex or caste of the students, but whoever learns something in any way is consider the student or person getting the education. Formal education is not the real education, but informal education cannot be considered to be unimportant. In practical life, one has to learn various kinds of education without which he cannot get success. There are two kinds of education, namely, the formal and informal. These two types of education are not substitute to each other but rather complement. Between formal, informal, incidental and intentional ways of education, there should always be a kind of balance. Undue importance should not be given to any kind of educational mode. There should be a kind of co-ordination between different kinds of educational means. As is understood till now that schools are not the only institution which provides education to individuals, but there are many agencies to impart such knowledge. There should be a kind of balance in all the institutions, otherwise, it is not possible to develop the individual in all the respects.

There are various experts belonging to this school of thought, which has provided various kinds of views on the concept of education. Some of the views of some experts are as follows —

In the words of Dumvile : Education in its wider sense consists of all the effects or influences which fall upon an individual during his passage from cradle to the grave.

In the words of S.S. Mackenzie : In the wider sense,

education is a process that goes on throughout life, and is being prompted by almost every experience in life.

In the words of Edward Thring : Education is the transmission of life by the living to the living.

NARROW VIEW OF EDUCATION

As said earlier, there is also a narrow view to see the concept of education. In this sense, education is a kind of training which takes place for a limited period of time. This period is confined to a restricted span of time. According to this school of thought, only the formal education is considered to be education. That education which is provided through a set curriculum, within a certain period of time and at a specific place is the education in real sense. This kind of education takes place only in school buildings.

In this kind of thinking, undue importance is provided to the schools. Schools are the only agency which provide education to all the human beings. In a school, education is being imparted directly and in a systematic manner and this kind of education is the only education in real sense. Schools are created or established with the only aim of providing formal kind of education to the child during the formative years and this procedure continues to a limited age. After getting this kind of education, one receive some degree, diploma or certificate, which proves that the human being has got education in formal manner in the school.

Today, various kinds of changes can be seen in every field and field of education is also not an exceptional case. In this field also, schools are now awarded with an important place and this view is supported with this school of thought.

Various experts have defined concept of education in narrow sense in the following manner :—

According to John Dewey : Schools exist in order to provide a special kind of environment for the formative years of human life.

According to S.S. Machenzie : In narrow sense, education can be taken to mean any well directed efforts to develop and cultivate our powers.

However, this ways of viewing the concept of education seems to be misleading because of the fact that there are various persons in our country as well as throughout the world who has not received higher educations, but still are very popular and successful persons in their lives. For instance, master blaster Sachin Tendulkar has got no higher level degrees but still he is very successful cricketer. Late Shri Dhiru Bhai Ambani was not very educated man, but a very successful businessman. Thus it can be said that this is not only formal education which matters in ones life, but informal education also plays an important role in the lives of individuals.

From the above discuss it can be said that education is not limited to the formal instructions which are being imparted in any school, but it also includes various kinds of experiences or learning which generate from the other informal agencies. It can be said that narrow meaning of education does not reflect the whole or complete process of education, but it is with the help of wider or broader view of education that we can get proper meaning of education.

As said earlier that with the time and development, various kinds of changes take place in various fields. This kind of changes take place because outlook of people gets changed. With the span of time and with the process of development, view of seeing or analysing the concept of education has also changed. The concept of education was different in ancient times in our country, it is different in modern time and different in other countries of the world. It is necessary to discuss all these aspects differently, which is as follows :—

ANCIENT INDIAN CONCEPT OF EDUCATION

Earlier in our country, people used to spend a very simple kind of life. Necessities of the peoples were very limited and they used to live a very peaceful life. As no much competition was there, people used to spent their more time in spiritual works or functions. Every field of life was influenced by spiritual thoughts. To a very great extent, concept of education was also influenced by these spiritual thoughts. During that time, education through Vedas was being imparted in which much importance was being provided to chastity, perseverance and independent thinking. Fundamental means of education were devotion, action and knowledge.

According to Upanishads education is considered to be a process resulting in achievement of salvation. Rig Veda consider the education as a process which helps to becomc a person selfless and self-reliant. Generally, various Gurus used to impart the education and all have different means to do this task. The concept of education in ancient times can be represented more clearly with the help of some of the views of these Gurus, which are as follows :—

According to Yajnavalkya, end result of the education is development of character of an individual with the help of which he becomes useful for the world.

According to Manu : There is no difference with a man without education and an animal.

According to Shankracharya : Process of education helps in producing self-realisation.

Thus, on the basis of above discussion and views provided by experts, it can be said that in ancient time, means to impart education were different and the objectives of the education at that time were also different. Education was considered one of an important means to make a human being different from animals.

NEW INDIAN CONCEPT OF EDUCATION

Because of various kinds of developments, one can easily analyse different kinds of changes in all the fields in our country, but in the field of education, no much changes has taken place. Modern educationists's thoughts reflect or are being affected by religion to a lot of extent. Even today, religion is considered the fundamental core of education. There are various experts who have provided their views on the concept of education, some of which are as follows :—

In the words of Vivekananda : Education is nothing but a manifestation of divine perfect which already exists in a man.

In the words of Tagore : Education unables a man to find out that ultimate truth which emancipates us from the bondage or restrictions of dust and provides the wealth of love and inner light.

In the words of Auribindo Ghose : Education is a process which helps in growing a person's soul to draw out that already exists within him.

WESTERNIZED CONCEPT OF EDUCATION

Greek philosophers and scholars influenced the

concept of education in west countries to a lot of extent. Plato is one of an important Greek philosopher and he recognizes process of education which continues throughout the life of human beings. Education not only provides knowledge, but it also develops innate values, and habits in an individual.

According to Plato, education should be such that it develops a kind of reason in the life of children so that they may can feel a harmony between soul and the various things existing in the world.

Plato considered harmony a true virtue. Educational system of Plato was based on moral education. One of an important educational principle of his system was virtues. He also regarded the virtues as essentials of universe. Truth, goodness and beauty were the foundations on which doctrine of Plato was based. Plato thought that only two forms of education can exist. The first kind of education enables a man to perform his daily activities and also make his sufficient to get knowledge to his aptitude. Second kind of education makes a man worthy of various kinds of state services.

Views of Plato are still considered to be the foundation of educational system of Western countries however, now some kinds of changes or variations can be seen.

Another important philosopher who has influenced the western concept of education is Aristotle. Aristotle consider education as a means to create a sound mind in a sound body. He said that education can develop man's faculty with the help of which he can enjoy the supreme truth and beauty.

In addition to both these experts, there are other philosophers also who have influenced the western concept of education to a lot of extent, some of which are as follows:—

In the words of G.H. Thompson : Education implies to adapt an individual in new or changing environment so that he can make invaluable contribution to human life in accordance to his utmost capacity.

In the words of R.R. Rusk : The main objective of education is to make a child so able that he can reconcile himself to reality in all its manifestations, not only to adopt himself to a natural environment.

In the words of Aldous Huxley : Education which trains up every human being to fit into the place one is to occupy in the social hierarchy should be considered a perfect education. However, in this process, one's individuality should not be destroyed in any way.

GOALS OF EDUCATION

The final output which is being got from the process of education is termed as its objective. Around a centre of purpose, an objective revolves. It is abstract in nature and can never realized fully. Process of education should be such that it can provide a kind of challenge to teachers and students as well. It should have the power to inspire towards greater effort.

Objective of education can be considered a hub of wheel, around which all other aims of education revolve or lie. It can be compared to a thread that can bring all valid objectives of education into an integrated form. Various experts have provided their views on the objectives of education, some of which are as follows :—

According to Swami Vivekanada : A perfect man making should be the objective of all kinds of education. Education, with the help of which character can be formed, strength of mind can be increased and intellect can be expanded should be taught.

According to Swami Dayananda : To lead towards liberation through development of character should be the ultimate objective of education.

According to Annie Besant : Aim of education should be to draw-out the child's innate capacities, and develop them in such a manner that he proves to be a useful, and healthy member of the society.

According to Gandhi Ji : Education which can draw out and stimulate the spiritual, intellectual and physical faculties of the children should be considered a true education.

To deal with various issues or aspects relating to education in our country, an commission, with the name Secondary Education C mmission was set up in the year 1952-53. The commission has mentioned four main objectives of education in India. According to the list provided by this commission, objectives of education include the following :—

a. Improvement of vocational efficiency,

b. Development of democratic citizenship,

c. Development of qualities for leadership, and

d. Development of personality.

In 1986, a New Policy of Education was prepared, in which goals of the education were mentioned very clearly. According to this policy, major goals of education are the following :—

a. To achieve an overall development of an individual with the help of integrated programme of education, and

b. To make education system such that it can play an important role in process of development of nation.

MAJOR OBJECTIVES OF EDUCATION

There lies a difference in the goals and objectives. Objectives are more specific statement of purpose in comparison to aims. If they are not remote, they are not abstracted also. It can be said that aims which are drawn or constructed for a short period of time are termed objectives. Thus, objectives are narrower than aims and they form an integral part of the whole.

Various experts have provided their opinion on the concept of objectives of education.

In the words of John Pestalozzi : Main objective of education is to develop and not to just to impart.

According to Indian Education Commission : The most important change needed in education is to transform it to relate it to the life, requirements and aspirations of the people, with the help of which education can be used as an important and powerful tool of social, economic and cultural transformations. Such kinds of transformations are necessary for realisation or fulfilment of national goals.

Health, worthy use of leisure, citizenship, ethical character, worthy home membership, command of fundamental processes and vocation are considered to be the major objectives of education by American Commission on the Reorganisation of Education, which was being set up in the year 1918.

From the above discussion it can be said that objectives of the education are related to different aspects of man's life. It is because of the reason that education is meant for the human beings.

Education has various broad objectives, which can be fulfilled or can be achieved with the help of certain policies and these policies should be used very cautiously and safely.

PLACE OF EDUCATION IN MODERN TIMES

We are living in the twentieth century and this period is considered to be the greatest transitional period in the history of mankind. Today, we see various kinds of changes being taking place in all the fields. Such changes have taken place with such a pace and in such a limited period of time that human beings do not get much time to adapt themselves in changing conditions.

Today, needs and requirements of human beings have increased to a lot of extent and education helps to a lot of extent in fulfilling these increasing needs and demands. All the changes taking place in the society or in all the spheres of life should be taken into account in education. It is necessary that education should have such programmes or policies which can prepare human beings for various changes.

With the development, various kinds of changes have also brought various kinds of problems and tensions. One of an important role education should play is to provide a kind of safeguard for all these tensions and problems. We are living in a technological age and to face various kinds of requirements, education plays an important role. Human beings can get the knowledge about the experiences of other human beings through the means of education. Today life has become very complicated and to solve out these problems, proper solution should be provided to human beings. These solutions are being provided by the education. What kind of important role education plays in the life of human beings, can be measured from the fact that today there is no aspect or field of life which is not affected by education.

From the following points, one can estimate the importance of education in modern era :

a. Development of inner powers and natural abilities: Human behaviour is influenced by various factors, such as love, affection, reasoning, imagination, curiosity etc. These natural inborn abilities can be developed and directed properly with the help of education.

b. Development of moral characters : Some experts consider character as destiny. Destiny of the nation is being built on the character. If people are lacking in character and moral values, it is not possible to reach greater heights. Education is an important agency which help in strengthening or building moral values and it helps in building up a strong character.

c. Development of all-round Personality : With the help of education, a man gets developed in all the respects. A balanced development takes place in the personality of human being with the help of education.

d. Modification in Environment : The society in which human beings live keeps on changing. Because of change in the society, the living environment also gets changed and every human being have to adapt himself to live in such a changed environment. An individual becomes able to adjust himself in changed environment with the help of education. According to the changing needs and requirements, one can also become able to mould the environment himself.

e. Base of whole life : A country is made up of its people and today's children will become citizens in the future.

As the child gets mature, he has to enter into new fields where he face new kind of problems. In this kind of life, he has to face various kinds of challenges and education makes a man able to face these kinds of challenges. Such kind of challenges have to be faced very courageously by the human beings and education prepares a man to face them successfully.

f. Encouragement of Social Development : With the education, a child gets the motivation to generate or learn the social ideals. With the education, his interest shifts towards the social services. There are some traits which are required to be learnt by all the individuals to become good social animal and these traits can be learnt by education very easily.

g. Fulfilment of Necessities : No one can lead a happy life with the fulfilment of some of the fundamental or basic needs or necessities. It is not very easy to fulfil such needs and education helps a man to learn those skills which can help him in satisfying his fundamental needs.

h. Provide Vocational Efficiency : The basic aim of all kinds of education is to provide the individual with such skills which can help him in getting a good job or make him able to become self-dependent. It is with the help of education only that a person can get a profession degree and establish his career as a profession.

i. Helps in Developing the Nation : A nation is composed of its citizens and if the citizens are well educated, standard or status of such nation will automatically increase to higher ranks. Thus it can be said that education helps in developing the nation. It can be said in other words that fundamental stone for national development is education.

j. Development of Religious Tolerance : We know that in India, various people of different caste and creed lives. In such kind of country where people follows different kinds of religions, it is not possible to maintain a kind of co-ordination among people unless and until people respects the religion of other people. Education helps in broadening the outlook of people which provides them with the ability to respect the values of other's religion.

Thus, we see that education plays an integral role not only in the modern era, but also in the ancient time also. Although some people consider education as a limited time process, but it is more justified to approach education as a whole life time procedure.

2

PHYSICAL EDUCATION—MEANING, AIMS AND OBJECTIVES

INTRODUCTION

Today's education not merely deals with mental enhancement of an individual, but also a source of physical activities that leads to all-round development of an individual. The best individual is one who is physically fit, mentally sound and sharp, emotionally balanced and socially well adjusted. It is therefore, 'physical education' said to be an integral part of 'Total Education'.

Generally physical education is misunderstood as merely physical activities or merely Mass physical training or just drill. It is important to overcome this misconception of physical education. The newly born discipline of physical education should be put into proper perspective and thoroughly studied for the welfare of the humanity at large. The importance of physical education and activity was recognized by Plato when he said "Lack of activity destroys the good conditions of every human being, while movement and methodical physical exercise save it and preserve it".

In establishing the position of physical education in the pattern of general Education it is important to present the brief role of physical Education in the past. Physical Education got its real existence in Greece- generally thought to be the first nation of the Europe to become utilized. This was really the first nation to give serious thinking and direction to educate and physical Education. The tiny states earlier GREECE had belligerent attitudes. As far as history of physical Education in GREECE is considered, the earlier GREECE can be divided into Four periods (1) period (2) Spartan period (3) Early Athenian period. (4) Later or Golden period.

World famous epics, Iliad and Odyssey proved importance of physical Education in Homeric age. Physical Education was not organized well but popular in social and political life. Chariot races, wrestling, foot races, shooting, dancing were activities famous in Greek. In 800 B.C - 700 BC History of Physical Education in Sparta gave clear indication that physical activities were regular for an individual. All round development of any person is well defined by Spartans. Spartans were called city soldiers and here aim of education confined to "Man of Action". Therefore Spartans mainly aims of Military Excellence were mainly accessed through regular and well-planned physical Educational programmes. In Early Athenian period, democratic approach was present but military importance was never underestimated. In leisure time physical activities were enhance and in the period, aim of Education was to develop. Body and mind harmoniously and proportionately. Physical activities were integral part of daily activities for every individual there. PALESTRA and DIDASCALEUM were the main institution of Education and physical education. Numerous Athletic celebrations were very famous. These celebrations traditionally known as ' Pan Hellenic games' were mainly dedicated to different Goods, such as Ancient 'Olympic' is for 'Zeus Pythian games' was dedicated to ' APOLLO' Isthmian Games' was dedicated to 'God of sea'. This shows the value of physical activities in social lives of Early Athenian People. In 'later Athenian Period' where individualism became the order of the day, emphasis was mainly laid on individual's personality development through physical education programs. Later Athenian Period has great contribution in new concepts of physical education by introducing new and modified subjects for enhancement of individual's personality such as 'Medical Gymnastics' natural diet programs and other fitness subjects. New approaches of analyzing fitness components were introduced and well planning was made on it. Similarly history of 'Rome' also displays the importance of physical education for those people which were said to be conservative. It was mainly thought that the physical vigor is necessary for rise of empire. In early Rome physical activities were actually introduced to improve skills for wars, as war was their chief occupation. Nobel families feel glad in participating dance activities. Dance activities were their integral event. Famous gladiatorial combats (264 B.C) another example showing the value given by Ancient society to this integral part of Education.

As human being took birth, body movements give first indications of beings fitness, therefore its nothing wrong in saying ' physical activity' plays an important part in human beings life all along. Since from primitive man to modern individual physical activities are necessary.

Meaning of Physical Education

The term physical Education consists of two separate

words, 'Physical and Education' .The first word 'Physical' is said to be related with bodily functions. Physical is relating to body or all the bodily characteristics. The term Physical may include the body functions, like digestive function, circulatory function or muscular function of any body, and it may be physical strength, physical endurance of any human being. In other words this word deals with fitness components and bodily effectiveness of any individual that can also be said as physical appearance.

The term 'Education' is described as a process in which and by which knowledge, character and behaviour of the individuals are understood and shaped. It is a systematic instruction for any particular task. Education is basically a preparation for life. Education is a training to learn and to apply that learning in real life. A combined meaning of these two words would be that systematic instructions and training which relate to physical activities or programme of activities, necessary for development of physical powers or cultivation of physical skill.

Education is not confined to any particular place. It is 'ever on' process. Education is a doing phenomenon also. Education can exist anywhere and any time. Same applied for Physical Education as well, A well planned and prepared process in physical education leads to healthful living. This not only increases physical efficiency of an individual but also social adoptability. Physical education is that part of education that cannot be neglected at any cost. This process leads to many quality development programmes which ultimately assist individual to become well social being. This educational process results in being vigorous and strong, with all due importance to mental health and emotion .In other words physical education for all around development of an individual. This means physical education covers all the aspects of physical, mental and social well being.

PHYSICAL EDUCATION ENABLE INDIVIDUALS TO MAINTAIN THEIR BODILY CONDITIONS IN THE BEST WORKING ORDER WITH ENHANCEMENT OF OTHER QUALITIES OF EFFICIENCY

Following points are making the concept of physical Education clearer.

(i) PHYSICAL EDUCATION IS AN EDUCATIONAL PROCESS

Physical education can no longer be treated as separate entity. Physical education cannot be separated from educational process. It is therefore said to be an integral part of total process of education. It is education of students through physical movements. Mind has no existence without body. Therefore physical education process is essential to fulfil the general aim of Education. Physical Education is that education which starts with physical development and advances towards perfect development of human being. Educational process has no existence with merely General Education, as just being intellectual is not the ultimate aim of this process, rather all round development is the real demand of educational process, and therefore one can not neglect physical Education from General Educational processes.

(ii) PHYSICAL EDUCATION DEALS WITH BIG MUSCULAR ACTIVITIES OR MOVEMENT EXPERIENCES

An individual gets movement experiences by involving himself/herself in Muscular activities. Any activity or task we perform, muscular movements are needed. In physical Education special attention is given on these muscular movements. Even if any human bring is in sleep one or the other muscle works (cardiac muscle). Physical education give us the experiences of muscular movements through different- different physical activities, the different activities lead human being to develop their physical standard. Though those big muscular activities the total personality of individuals is developed. Any skill in the field of Sports and Games is mainly dependent on the muscular movement of performer. The sequential movement of performer depends on skill acquisition and other learning methods. Physical Education deals with these learning methods and assists performer to perform good muscular movements that lead to good health of individuals. To give more experience of muscular activities, physical education programme includes essential subjects like anatomy, physiology, kinesiology or Bio/Mechanics etc.

(iii) RESPONSES GAINED THROUGH MOVEMENT EXPERIENCES

Just experiencing "Big Muscular Activities" is not an end in physical Education. The responses gained after this movement experiences is the essential part of learning process. These responses actually make our life more efficient and bring perfection in performance that ultimately leads us to Good skills and healthy life. Analyzation of any activity learned is must, the incorrect performance must be corrected and practiced again and again. The more the individuals get experience of movements more responses will be gained. Responses are actually the perfection gained by an individual. These responses teach to respond in a healthful way to increase demand placed on them through gained responses individual develop great endurance and be able to perform his duty according to his capacity with well adjusted and skilled manner. The quality of keeping fit is essential for leading a happy, vigorous and abundant life. These responses can be taken in two different aspects:-

(a) Physical fitness/organic development/skills

(b) Mental skills moral or social development

(a) Physical fitness/organic development/skills improvements.

On the one hand the responses gained through movement experiences leads to physical power for the individual. Individual gets control over the motor mechanism of human body that means individual is well capable to analyze his/her own movements and he/she have the ability to cut down waste motions. Individual can now make judgments and interpret situations correctly. The responses lead to develop physical fitness components and individual gets more body control and efficiency in movements.

(b) Mental skills, moral or social development.

Apart from organic development or physical fitness, responses gained through movement experiences assists in development of mental skills of an individual. The movement experiences in physical education do not only lead to physical fitness of an individual, this experience also enhances the mental capability. Physical education make individual to experience social values through physical activities. Individual gets the qualities of well social being. Through the responses, individual not only learn physical skills or co-ordination but must acquire knowledge such as rules, techniques cooperation. All individuals must know about their body, importance of sanitation, factors in disease prevention, importance of exercise, need of balanced diet etc. The store of new knowledge will equip an individual to interpret new situations. As a result of participation in activities the individual will be able to draw conclusions himself. Therefore individual will be able to take wise decisions too. By learning the skills of adjustment through the experiences of body movements, the quality of social adaptability is developed. Situational learning's in Physical activities lead to increase this quality more. When these muscular movements are performed in a group or individuals new work as a team, the experience develop the responses of group consciousness and cooperative living. Developing of these social desirable traits is basic concern of an ideal programme of physical Education.

In real words the experiences gained through 'big muscular activities' and the related responses of these experiences leads to 'All round development' of an individual. The qualities developed in an individual through physical Education are very valuable for the society, which no doubt enhances nations proud and ultimately work for the MANKIND.

DEFINING PHYSICAL EDUCATION

Acceptance of any particular definition depends upon the thinking of that particular physical Educator. One definition of physical Education may not be enough to explain the discipline completely. It also means different things to different people. Apart from the wide concept of physical education the problem lies upon the misunderstanding of this discipline. In General words it is said that physical Education is whatever physical Educators do. Therefore the acceptance or non-acceptance of any particular definition lies on the ideas of Evaluators. Throughout the History, Physical Education has been misunderstood. More often it has been confused with physical training, Games, play etc. But as we go deep into this discipline, we find that physical Education is must more than merely these terminologies. Different physical Educationists have given different definitions. Definitions of some reckoning physical Educationists are given below:-

"Physical Education is that phase of the whole field of education that deals with big muscles activity and their related responses."

— J.B. Nash

"Physical Education is an integral part of total Education process is a field of endeavourer, which has its aim. The development of physically, Mentally, Emotionally and socially fit citizen through the Medium of physical activities, which has been reflected with a view to realizing these outcomes."

— Charles A. Bacher.

"Physical Education is the sum of man's physical activities. Selected as to kind and conducted as to outcomes."

— J.F. William

"Physical Education is Education through physical activities for the development of total personality of the child and its fulfilment and perfection in body, mind and spirit."

— J.P. Thomas

"Physical Education is the accumulation of wholesome experiences through participation in large muscles activities that promote optimum growth and development."

—Brownhill and Hagman

"Physical Education is the sum of changes in the individual caused by experiences involving in motor activity."

— R. Cassidy

"Physical Education is a way of Education through Motor activities and related experiences and its subject matter is primarily related with the ways of behaving."

— William H.Kilpatrick

"Physical Education is a way of education through physical activities which are selected and carried on with full regard to values in human growth, development and behaviour."

—A.A. H.P.E.R

"Physical Education is the accumulation of wholesome experiences through participation in large muscle activities that promote optimum growth and development."

—Brownwell

"Physical Education is an indispensable part of all health programmes. Its various activities should be so planned as to develop the physical and mental health of the students, cultivate recreational interest and skills, and promote the spirit of team work, sportsmanship and respect for others, Physical Education is therefore, must more than drill or a series of regulated exercise. It includes all forms of physical activities and games, which promote the development of the body and the mind.'

—Secondary Education Commission Report

"Physical Education is that part of education which has to do with the development and training of the whole individual through physical activities."

— A.R. Wayman

— A.Are. Vamen

"Physical Education is the sum of those experiences which come to the individual through movement."

—Delbert Obertwuffer

"Physical Education is the social process of change in the behaviour of the human organism, Originating primarily from the stimulus of social- big muscle- play and related activities.

—Charer. C. Cowell

"Physical Education is that part of the general education programme which is concerned with the growth, development and education of children through the medium of big-muscle activities. It is education of the whole child by means of physical activities. Physical activities are the tools. They are so selected and conducted as to influence every aspect of child's life physically, mentally, emotionally and morally."

—H.C. Buck

"Physical Education is that phase of the whole process of education which is concerned with vigorous muscular activities and related responses and with the modification in the individual resultant from these responses."

—Nexon and Cozen

"Physical Education is education through physical activities for the development of the total personality of the child, to its fullness and perfection in body, mind and spirit. Immediately, it is concerned with the development of physical fitness. In striving for such fitness, however, physical education has to train the child's mental, moral and social qualities, arouse its awareness of environment and develop alertness, presence of mind, resourcefulness, discipline, cooperation and the spirit of respect, sympathy and generality towards others- qualities that are essential for a happy and well adjusted life in a free and democratic world. Physical education can thus, make a very valuable contribution to our national life."

—A national plan for physical Education and Recreation. A report by Ministry of Education Govt of India.

AIMS, OBJECTIVES AND SCOPE OF PHYSICAL EDUCATION

General aim of physical Education is:

1. All round development of an individual.

The steps or process to get the aim 'All-round development of individual' are the general objectives of physical education. Below are mentioned the general objectives of physical education:-

- ➢ Organic vigour
- ➢ Neuro muscular development
- ➢ Personality development

- Good personal Habits
- Useful living.

(i) ORGANIC VIGOUR

Physical Education includes physical activities programmes that make the individual physically healthy and fit. Good physical fitness programmes making all body system efficient and more stimulated. Physical activities includes various games and sports, mass demonstration activities like calisthenics, Rhythmic Gymnastics, Bhartium, Marching and drills etc. which are really influential and very effective in making individual physically fit.

Systems like digestive, respiratory, crematory etc. becomes more efficient as all directly or indirectly influenced positively by performing regularly and systematically in physical activities. Influence of physical activities on Muscular system is clearly visible. In short all biological or physiological and anatomical systems or every organ used in these becomes more productive.

Apart from physical activities physical educational programmes provide every knowledge to keep oneself fit and productive. Subjects like health Education, Nutritional Education, six education, sports physiology etc. are no doubt very beneficial for preventing harms of various kinds like injuries communicable diseases, food poisoning etc. which assist individual to stay fit and keep the organs well functional.

(ii) NERO MUSCULAR DEVELOPMENT

Nero muscular system is the functional coordination between Nervous system and muscular system. This means batter body movements. Physical Education programmes leads to development of skills. Good functioning of body systems and mental alertness comes out through very actuate and skillful movements. Activeness of individual and timely execution of movement leads to better task performance. Physical Education having objective of efficient performance of movement leads to better task performance. Physical Education having objective of efficient performance of movements or performance of good skills with the expenditure of required energy only. This Nero-muscular coordination improves the body control, makes body movements very graceful and effective .In other words physical Education deals with mental preparedness apart from good physical out put.

(iii) PERSONALITY DEVELOPMENT

One of the major objectives of physical Education is personality Development. Activities and other educational programmes assist in needed behavioural changes in an individual. Physical education not only improves fitness aspect of the personality but also works for development of social qualities. Physical Education helps to create good personality individuals with all possible socially acceptable behavioural qualities like cooperation, good character, self-control, leadership qualities etc. Physical activities helps individual to improve his behaviour socially acceptable and therefore objectives of creating good social being can easily achieved through participation in Games and sports or other physical activities.

(iv) GOOD PERSONAL HABITS

Good habits always exist to lead good life style. Personal habits like good utilization of leisure time, timely taking food (meals), appropriate sleeping duration, playing habits, regular workout (energy expenditure) not using alcohol etc. physical education aware individual about good habits and motivates and adopt these habits. For effective and productive personality good personal and socially acceptable habits are essential. Good habits helps in over coming body deformities, infections, diseases, wrong or negative thinking which ultimately produces good social beings.

(V) USEFUL LIVING

Healthy and fit human being is effective or productive only if, he/she is useful to mankind. Physical Educational activities tell the ways to make life more useful. Human being is called social being only of he/she is productive for society. Loyalty for Nation, wellness of others, and helping and cooperating team-mates is essentially needed for development of Nation. In other words physical Educational programmes produces needed qualities in individuals which too assists in creating all round development of human being.

2. Following paints are also required as objectives of physical Education which ultimately leads for whole some **development of Individuals for complete living.**

3. American Association for health, physical Education and Recreation (AAHPER) has presented for objectives of physical Education which re listed below:

(i) Skilful Movements- Physical Education helps children to move in a skilled and effective manner in all relative activities in which they are engaged through the activities in physical Education.

(ii) Knowledge of Related scientific principles- Physical Education help children to understand and appreciate scientific principles of concerning movements so that their have proper utilization of these knowledge in life style.

(iii) Better relationships- Physical education help children to development of better interpersonal relationships.

(iv) Good functional organs- Physical education help children to develop the various organic systems of the body, so that they respond in a healthful way to the increased demand placed on them.

SCOPE OF PHYSICAL EDUCATION

An extent to what any discipline can reach is said to be the scope of that particular discipline. Physical Education having very wide scope, it is not limited to mere physical activities or physical exercises. Physical education include every aspect that lead individual to all round development. History of various Nations has proved physical Education is in cultural heritage of human beings. Physical Education is not limited to school or college curricular but has successfully influenced human beings in all walk of life, and in every field of development. Age, sex or physical abilities of individuals have no bar as far as physical educational programmes are concerned.

Scope of physical Education covers following:-

- Games and sports
- Corrective exercises
- Basic stances and exercises
- Rhythmic activities/programmes
- Social Awareness programmes
- Educational institution curriculum

- Scientific Methodology
- Rehabilitative programmes

(ii) Games and sports

Games and sports widen the scope of physical Education to extreme. It includes every fame of football, cricket soccer chess etc.

(Team game , individual game) or in other words it includes any variety of game or sport e.g. combative, ball game, indigenous etc. physical Education has its influence in every part of it. Any skill display includes physically Education; Physical itself clears its scope in this field, but this merely not the knowledge of physical activities. The load planning, the intensity of sports activity, playing technique, tactics and making of strategies all includes effective educational processes given by physical education. Therefore Games and sports cannot be taken apart from its scope.

(ii) Corrective Exercises and Rehabilitative programme

Good posture makes individual work efficiently. This knowledge of correct and good basic posture is presented effectively by physical Educationist. Even a wrong sitting habit can lead to bad posture, many times work demands results in bad posture, physical education clears the basic concept about the posture and presents the effective exercises to overcome bad postures.

(iii) Basic stances and Exercises

Every productive skill needs good and accurate position of the athlete. Physical Education introduces to us different exercises for different skills for better performance. Knowledge about the stances, grips, action and execution of the skills assists in enhancing the performance. Therefore physical education has its effective and successful scope in the field of physical Education.

(iv) Recreational programmes

Today's world every individual needs to recharge oneself to become more productive even after heavy workload. Physical Educational processes include Recreational activities as its essential programme. After the heavy work out every human wants to feel relaxed and recreational, physical Education introduces many Recreational activities that refreshes and recharges the individual. This scope of physical Education on the other hand contributing a lot in mankind.

(v) Rhythmic Activities

Rhythmic activities include folk dances, aerobics, lezium etc. which mainly enhances the coordinative ability of an individual. We cannot neglect the fact that many of these Rhythmic Activities is integral part of our Indian culture like Bhangra and other folk dances. Therefore it is validly said that physical Education is in cultural heritage of India.

(vi) Social Awareness programmes

Physical Education introduces us about Hygiene, sex education, prevention from injuries etc. which ultimately proves very assisting to society.

(vii) Educational Institutions curriculum

Educational institutions having physical activities as essential part of curriculum. This mainly includes 'INTRAMURAL AND EXTRAMURAL PROGRAMMES" physical training through activities like calisthenics, Bhartium and other mass training exercises clears the wide scope of physical Education.

(viii) Scientific Methodology

Bio-mechanics, sports physiology, sports science, sports psychology etc. newly introduced subjects in the field of physical Education widens its scope in the scientific field of Education. Every day new methodology is being introduced for the enhancement of sports field. The urge to grow faster and achieve new heights in the field of sports no doubt increasing the scope of physical Education.

(ix) Rehabilitative programme

For temporary-injured athlete it is very important to maintain his/her fitness level. Physical education widen its scope by introducing Rehabilitative exercises which aims to reduce the recovery period of injured athlete and also maintains the fitness components (strength, speed, endurance, flexibility etc.) that ultimately leads for better performance after recovery).

(x) Coaching

The wide scope of physical education also covers Coaching. In the field of Coaching knowledge of physical education makes coaches more empowered and efficient. Many basic aspects of coaching is easily understood by the physically educationists and the theoretical subjects matter as well as practical aspects are widely covered in Physical education.

MODERN CONCEPT OF PHYSICAL EDUCATION

The modern concept of physical Education does not refer physical Education as military exercises or limited to physical counting exercises. The new concept of physical dedication is not at all concluding physical education as a drilling marching programme or enjoying only with some sort of mass displaying activities. Modern concept of physical education is well emphasized, understood and recognized in the existing society. Following are explained modern approach and trends in physical education.

1. Philosophical approach

In the modern era physical education has been accepted as a wide philosophical approach, which is individual, as well as society centered. New every individual and society as a whole has understood the social valves in physical education. It is no more misunderstood as limited to parade grounds or gymnasiums. Modern concept emphasized physical education as a influencing source of developing positive and progressive thinking in the society.

2. Education process

Modern concept of physical education refers physical activities as an Education approach. Physical activities present as many education values not limited to body development only. Physical education also involves education process as other general educational subjects. In modern era physical education is highly accepted, recognized and implemented in schools, colleges and universities.

3. Professional Approach

Earlier no specific profession courses were preferred in the field of physical Education. A Military or sports background was enough to engage in the profession. Modern concept of physical education provide specific professional approach through specified courses like B.P.Ed/ B.P.E, M.P.Ed /M.P.E and related Diploma's courses.

4. Scientific Approach

Modern concept of physical education is much scientific in nature. Physical education is now more empowered with new subjects of sports medicine, sport Biomechanics, sport psychology etc. new approaches of Researches and analysations have changed the old concept of physical education and these approaches clearly indicates the importance of physical education in every walk of life for every individual.

5. New trends and methodologies adopted

Misconception of physical education, that it is limited to drills and exercises is completely rejected. New trends and methodologies like rhythmic exercises, musical coordination's, rehabilitation exercises; yoga therapy, modern equipments and much more are being adopted by society. Every day new and more authentic theories or exercises methodology is existing and making physical education more and more valuable for individuals and society.

The modern concept of physical education leading to progression and development in the society.

IMPORTANCE AND NEED OF PHYSICAL EDUCATION IN SCHOOL/COLLEGE/SOCIETY

Following are mentioned the importance and need of physical education:

(i) Proper growth and development

Proper growth and development of child depends mainly upon the surrounding atmosphere. Physical Education provides opportunity to children's for their proper growth and development. Its very essential to develop habits which assist students to grow effectively. In other words physical Education is very essential for 'All round development of an Individual.'

(a) Physical development - Playing activities makes the child's anatomical and physiological systems progressive.

(b) Mental development- Physical activities are also helping children's to become mentally sharp and smart. Mentally preparing children for the future is definitely shows the importance of the discipline.

(c) Socially Acceptable- Playing situations teach children how to cooperate adjusts and manages in a group. This kind of development makes children more socialized.

(ii) Psychological development

Psychological development includes emotional stability, aggressiveness, and arousal etc. aspects. Physical Education in school age (teenagers) children's become psychologically confused many times. In order to have good development of psychological aspects physical education, which is said to be the best source for this, must be programmed properly and essentially in secondary schools.

(iii) Better Fitness level

Physical Education involves various physical exercise programmes for different age groups. Good fitness level sound mind lies in healthy body proves the importance of physical education in Secondary schools.

(iv) Healthy Environment

Grounds and fields are the basic requirements of physical Education. The presence of other facilities, equipments motivate children to live happy and use the facilities for the betterment. Open air, safety, playing with classmates makes environment very healthy.

(v) Providing knowledge

Physical Education is not limited to physical activities or mass drills. Apart from the knowledge of the field of Games and sports Physical education covers the valuable subjects like "Health Education, "Sports medicine, "Sports Psychology" Sports management, body physiology for which is really contributing a lot in making a healthful society. These subjects assist in learning skills to preventing diseases.

(vi) Leadership quality

Physical Education provides number of opportunities to every student to develop this quality. Playing the lead/ up games or any game of general nature helps in developing one or the other quality of leadership like confidence, cooperation, loyalty discipline etc. This assist the student to face challenges came in the future.

(vii) Interest of Students

Physical Education makes the education programmes more interesting. Good learning only takes place if one is interested for it. The recreational games and leaders activities create interest in child to learn with interest.

(viii) Acceptable Attitude

Attitude plays important role in ones personality. Mainly attitude is more influence in the adolescence age of any individual. Physical activities and learning processes teaches one the appropriate attitude against climates opponents, teachers, and parents.

(ix) Total personality

The physical development improvement of other behavioural aspects ultimately helps in producing good personality individuals. Psychological changes plays effective role in this. It is a also famous said that if you want to know ones personality, check first about the same individuals physical activities participation.

(x) Personal Habits

Using of Leisure time, good sitting and walking style, Balanced diet etc. are habits which lead to better life style. Physical Education motives students to be in good habits and productive for society.

(xi) Occupational Importance

Physical Education Health programmes are emerging as very demanding profession. Now a days every one is health conscious .It is therefore preferred by students to get every advantage from this discipline. They can also have this disciplines profession, which is really in interest of society.

(xii) National Integration

Working with others as a team is attractive characteristic of this field. Putting efforts together to score good or performing mass demonstration assist for national integration. To workout in a collative manner to achieve goals teaches the importance of integration. Every student must recognize value of integration.

(xiv) Creative approach

Every activity needs creativeness, the same applies in the field of physical Education. But this field gives more opportunities to put creative efforts practically on field. This makes individual more creative and confidant. For students this quality is required for facing real life situations effectively.

(xv) Democratic approach

Working with a cooperative and understanding manner on grounds naturally emphasized on democratic effort. Motivating every team member and moving ahead with each others suggestions. Formulating moves while playing any game in the best example of democratic approach. We received from the field of physical Education. It is required to let every student work in a democratic atmosphere.

Above given points clears us the need and importance of physical Education in secondary schools.

PROBLEMS EXIST WHILE ORGANISING PHYSICAL EDUCATION PROGRAMMES IN SCHOOLS AND COLLEGES

Note- To Easily Understand the Misconceptions about Physical Education This Topic is presented as the Problems in Organizing Physical Education Programme Schools and Colleges.

Physical education is essential and regular part of school total educational curriculum. Physical activities are needed to assist students in achieving total personality. With the new concept of physical education, this discipline is new no more limited to Games and sports only. The wide scope of physical education itself demands very specific concentration and effective planning. So that full advantages of it can be passed on to students. Unfortunately the field of physical Education still undergoing some misconceptions and these invalid aspects are hindrances in proper. Organizational planning of application of physical Education programmes. The proper application of curriculum needs practical awareness of real situations. Any kind of misunderstanding in analyzing effects and importance of any subject may result in ineffective curriculum set ups.

Therefore it is essential to highlight the problems existing while planning for regular physical education programmes in any educational institutions. Valid placement of subjects in school curriculum of any subject can make educational processes more effective and production. Below are given some common problems relative to the field of physical education in Indian schools or almost every educational institution.

(i) This subject 'Physical Education' is being misunderstood

Physical Education is misunderstood as games and drills only. The wide scope of physical education covers all aspects need for the development of an individual. Physical Education is not limited to sports fields only, it analysis the mechanical body movements, aware about the health components and touches many more scientific aspects. Because of this misunderstanding the discipline of physical education do not getting appropriate placement in regular school curriculum systematically.

(ii) Wastage of Time

Commonly the subject of physical education is wrongly considered as wastage of time. It is a general thought that the subjects like 'Math', 'Science', 'social Studies' etc. develops the aspects like intelligence, confidence etc. but not physical education. In reality physical education develops the wholesome personality of students more naturally. Therefore students are not preferred to waste their time in physical activities but to go for extra classes in other subjects. This is one of the main reasons that lead to improper organization of physical education programmes in educational institutions.

(iii) Wastage of Money

Games and reports, and even other subjects comes under Physical Education like sport- Biomechanics, sport-Medicine, sport training etc. require some general and specific equipments apparatus and facilities like play fields etc. which demands money. In the same side these equipments and facilities require proper and regular maintenance also. Many organizers considering as draw back and therefore rarely prefer this discipline Even some parapets also thinking the physical activities as money demanding only. This misconception also results in improper organization of physical education programmes.

(iv) Physical Education as profession

Very few students really go for physical education with motive to take it as profession. It is again question of misconception that Physical education gives very less opportunities to earn good amount with good social status. This makes the physical Education as less demanding subject by students and this also make organizers to put less effort for the proper implementation in School curriculum. But in the true side physical education is an integral part of total education programme and the demand for physical teachers increasing highly. Other institutions like health clubs, rehabilitative exercises, sports and games etc. too are in good demand of physical teachers/instructors.

v. Undiscipline in Education Institutions

Practical situations in rounds are totally different

comparing to classroom situations. Fields while playing some valid voices, talks are obvious but many think this behaviour of students as undiscipline. Off course creating undemanding noise, disturbing others, showing any kind of misbehaviour must be tactfully handled by physical education teacher. Mainly is through that the students that create undiscipline or those students who misbehave have chosen physical Education as subject. Therefore organizers also try not to introduce this subject. Proper and accurate planning is needed for productive placement of Physical Education in School curriculum.

vi. Weak Students

Organizers mainly worried about weak students and with the thinking that week students are only interested in games and sports, they give less attention on physical Education programme as a whole. This leads in giving less time period for physical activities to students and facing the weak students for studies. Organizers must give full attention to both the aspects (Physical as well as intellectual) for students and therefore must be given balanced schedule to students.

PLACE OF PHYSICAL EDUCATION IN THE GENERAL EDUCATION PROCESS

If the aim of Education is enrichment of personality, Physical Education contributes to much extent. If the aim of Education is self realization, again no doubt physical Education provides opportunities to develop the sense of self realization. To achieve and realize the aim and objectives of Education, physical Education plays an important role and assist in developing those objectives more practically. Therefore, it is said that physical education is an integral part of general education process.

Whole Educational processes become more easy and efficient when physical Education put its contributions. Physical education is an essential part of total education process. Secondary Education Commission (1952-53) enlisted four aims of education i.e.

(i) Development of democratic approach,

(ii) Improvement of vocational efficiency,

(iii) Development of personality and

(iv) Development of qualities of leadership.

Physical education puts its great contribution in developing these qualities in an individual.

Two statements 'A sound mind lies in a sound body' and 'physical Education an integral part of total Education', one statement empowers the other statement. A complete personality is consisted of healthy body and healthy mind. In other words it can be said physical education assist whole educational process in developing all round personality. Only theoretical approach may produce a sound mind, but for a sound body physical approach is required. Therefore only class room education itself cannot be considered as a complete educational programme until and unless physical education is regarded as an integral part of the programme. Relationship of physical education with general education is well recognized and understood. It is therefore, physical education found essentially place in regular curriculum of every education institution.

Following given points present, the importance and contributions of physical education in the total education process.

1. Interesting

Sports and games, recreation and other physical activities create interest in students and they become motivated to follow educational programmes. Physical Education makes education programme more interesting. Physical education is a source of recreation and relaxation. It keep students happy and enjoyable, which make students energetic and interesting in the total educational programmes.

2. Effective and Easy learning

Only classroom learning in educational programmes may not be much effective. Learning of social valves like cooperation, adjustment, teamwork, self-control etc. is more effective and practical in physical education. Student's participation in different physical activities provides ample opportunities to learn many educational valves. Therefore physical education assist total education programme in effective and easy learning of students.

3. Healthy approach

Physical education develops competitive spirit with a cooperative attitude. This aspect bring programme in the total education programme. Students try to perform their best in classrooms or in Examinations with a cooperative attitude. Apart from this, physical activities make students physically fit and mentally healthy. This can be concluded as physical education makes total education programme a healthy approach.

4. Responsibilities and Discipline

Physical Education through its various activities

assists in developing sense of responsibility and discipline in students. These qualities make possible the smooth and effective running of education programmes. Therefore, total education programme possibly achieve the motive of producing valuable citizens for the country.

5. Knowledge

Physical education coves wide range of subjects like Physiology, human anatomy, psychology, sport medicine, health education etc., which involve huge knowledge for the students. Learning of healthy education first aid, communicable diseases, diet and nutrition like topics is very essential for children's and adolescents. Updating of knowledge is one of the main objectives of any education programme. Physical Education contributes a lot also in relation to providing beneficial knowledge to students.

6. Growth and Development

During the phases of infant to adolescent individual requires special attention for their proper growth and development. Absence of any physical activities may harm the normal growth and development. In this stage students require some specific kind of physical activities, which assist in their growth and development. Education curriculum must be involving such activities for proper growth and development of students.

7. Friendship and Relationship

Sports and other physical activities provide an environment for every one to feel enjoyable and understand each other. Physical education assist in strengthening relationships and develop the quality of group dynamics. It improves student - student and student - teacher relationship. Good relations bring progress in the general education programme.

8. Other

Physical education develops many other such qualities behaviour or attitude that make physical education an important part of total education programme. Physical education develops leadership qualities and personal habits acceptable attitude with Creativeness in students.

Physical education therefore plays an important and arsenical role in the general education programme.

3

SOCIOLOGICAL FOUNDATION OF PHYSICAL EDUCATION

The sociology of education is the study of how social institutions and forces affect educational processes and outcomes, and vice versa. By many, education is understood to be a means of overcoming handicaps, achieving greater equality and acquiring wealth and status for all. Learners may be motivated by aspirations for progress and betterment. Education is perceived as a place where children can develop according to their unique needs and potentialities. The purpose of education can be to develop every individual to their full potential. The understanding of the goals and means of educational socialization processes differs according to the sociological paradigm used.

Education in its broadest sense is any act or experience that has a formative effect on the mind, character, or physical ability of an individual (e.g., the consciousness of an infant is educated by its environment through its interaction with its environment); and in its technical sense education is the process by which society deliberately transmits its accumulated knowledge, values, and skills from one generation to another through institutions. Teachers in such institutions direct the education of students and might draw on many subjects, including reading, writing, mathematics, science and history. This technical process is sometimes called schooling when referring to the compulsory education of youth. For example, Samuel Bowles and Herbert Gintis, Teachers in specialized professions such as astrophysics, law, or zoology may teach only a certain subject, usually as professors at institutions of higher learning. There is also instruction in fields for those who want specific vocational skills, such as those required to be a pilot. In addition there is an array of education possible at the informal level, e.g., at museums and libraries, with the Internet, and in life experience.

MEANING OF SOCIOLOGY AND SPORTS SOCIOLOGY

Meaning of Sociology

Sociology is the study of the individuals groups and institutions that make up human society. Sociology is a social science, which includes every aspect of human social conditions. It is a scientific study of social life and hence considered a social science.

The word sociology existed from combination of Latin word Socials means companion and logos means knowledge. Companion here refers to group of people or society and knowledge is to science to gain.

Sociology is the scientific study of society science of society sociology is a discipline, which provides us knowledge about various aspects of society.

The word sociology first cropped up in 1937 AD by French philosopher August Comte. According to August Comte, "Sociology is the field focuses on how and why people are organized in society, either as individuals or as groups. Sociology is said to be study of the relationship between the society and the individual."

SOME IMPORTANT DEFINITIONS OF SOCIOLOGY

Max Weber

"Sociology is a science which interprets social behaviour with the aim of arriving at a causal explanation of human behaviour."

"Sociology is the science, which attempts the interpretative understanding of social action."

F.Le Play

"Sociology is an observational science which studies social phenomena."

Park and Burges

"Sociology is the science of collective behaviour of beings."

J.F. Cuber

"Sociology is a subject of scientific knowledge of human relationships.

Rocek

"Sociology is one of the group of subjects classed as the social science, all of which describe the objective study of social experiences."

Moore and Cole

"Sociology studies the behaviour of the individuals which is performed in relation to the other individuals in society."

Giddings

"Sociology is a systematic description and explanation of society as a whole."

Gillin & Gillin

"Sociology is said to be the study of inter section arising from the association of living beings."

Sociology studies the social life of human beings. It is the science that examines human beings relationships with one another and with the society as a whole. Sociology studies the individual's actions and reactions as the member of society.

Following conclusion can be drawn from the above definitions and discussions.

i. Sociology is an academic and applied discipline that studies about society and its members.

ii. It involve all kind of social processes exist in society.

iii. Sociology examines analysis and evaluates every such aspect, which influence human beings in the society.

iv. Sociology deals with all social institutions, which directly or indirectly related with members of society.

v. Sociology is a scientific study of social interaction that takes place between the individual and society.

vi. Sociology is a study of human relations and its affects on individuals and society as a whole.

SPORT SOCIOLOGY

The subject sport sociology is concerned with a study of people, groups, communities, and other human activities in relation to sports. It is concerned with the social and individual behaviour with respect to the influences and reactions of physical activities and sports .As like the general concept of socialization sport sociology depends on the society and cultural heritage of individuals. In the field of physical education and sports sociology plays an important role to establish and develop sports behaviour. Sport sociology is a positive approach of the democratic way of life Sport sociology is concerned with a study of people and their institutions related with sports to establish better social order. Sports sociology plays an important part in solving social problems. Sport sociology improves the social behaviour of a social being through different approach under sports and physical education. Sports sociology aims for developing sports behaviour, helping in the development of healthy and physically fit individuals, developing an understanding of the worthy use of leisure time, developing and promoting the positive thinking in the society through sports and physical activities.

DEFINITIONS OF SPORT SOCIOLOGY

Sport sociology is the behavioural study of individual and society as a whole in relation to sports.

Sports sociology is an approach through which human society organizations, groups and individuals come under the influences of sports and physical activities.

Sports sociology is concerned with the study of people and their institutions related with sports.

Sport sociology is the behavioural study of groups/ teams, individual and society as a whole through physical activities, competitions and sports participations.

Sport sociology is an approach to develop sports behaviour through various physical activities and sports competitions.

Sport sociology is the sub-field of sociology, which deals with the study of society, its affects/influences on an individual or group through inter-relationships of sports with various elements of culture.

Sport sociology is a science, as well as art sociology is empirical science .it is a scientific discipline having its own methods of investigation like observation, interrogation, etc. sport sociology is based on collective wisdom and knowledge gathered from different schools of thought.

Sports sociology studies the relationship between sport and other factors of life, such as family, education, politics, and economy relation etc. sport sociology concerns about the social organizations, group behaviour and interaction patterns that exist in different types of sports. Spot sociology deals with the social processes that occur in conjunction with sport such as socialization, stratification, social change etc. it is a study of cultural structural and situational factors affecting sport and sport experiences.

IMPORTANCE OF SOCIOLOGY IN THE FIELD OF PHYSICAL EDUCATION

Sports are a physical activity occurs in a given cultural mailer and is socially structured. Human individual is a social being and he develop and prayers in society. An individual perform any physical activity or sports with in the society only. Any physical activity or sport that exists in society viewing its influences group or society. Therefore, physical education and sports cannot its influences on individuals.

It is the subject of sociology that helps us in understanding socialization. Socialization is a process by which individuals learn about their environment and acquire social characteristics.

On the one hand socialization can also be explained as a process of acquiring social values and living together on the other hand physical education and sports also deals with learning of social values and collective performances.

Therefore, sociology having great importance in the field of physical education and sports. Following are some importance in the filed of physical education and sports.

1. Sports as a Social Phenomena

Sociology focuses on sports as social phenomena. Influences of sports on an individual or society are importantly analyzed through various social aspects. Sociology deals with individuals, groups which also engaged in sports. Sociology helps in understanding every aspect of these social phenomena. It therefore helps in the upliftment and better understanding of sports in the society.

2. Sports Ethics

Sociology develops social valves in individuals or groups, which directly or indirectly enhances sports ethics in an athlete. An athlete is a social being; .He applies the learned social valves in sports and shows good sportsman spirit. In the filed of sports ethics (fair play, respect etc.) is highly required and sociology plays great role in it.

3. Role Play

The process of socialization teaches us "Role play" as an important aspect. Every social being is essentially comes under the aspect. Role-play. Realization and understanding the responsibilities by an individual makes the society healthy and more progressive.

Similarly in the filed of physical Education and sports 'Role-playing' learned through socialization is very important.

4. Quality Sports

Social valves, ethics status developed through socializations helps in providing us quality sports. For the development of physical education and sports, sociology assists in providing quality sports to society. Quality sports are the need of hour this can help in the development of the field of physical Education and sports.

5. Cooperation and Competition

Cooperation and competition are two important characteristics of socialization that exist in society. Sociology give importance to both aspects and in sports both exist together. Sociology teaches us that cooperation's as important as competition in society. Sports also required good and healthy relationship between competition and cooperation. Sociology aware us about their importance in society and in the field of physical education and sports.

6. Sports Become More Educative

Sociology makes sports and games more educative and valuable for the sports persons or society. Sociology teaches us social values and importance of healthy relationships, sports further strengthens the social values. It is not possible for any athlete to develop good cooperation and sportsmanship with out understanding social values. Hence, sociology plays important role in making sports more educative and valuable for the society.

7. Social Control and Self-Discipline

In the field of sports many times spectators go out of control and this may lead to heavy mass causalities. Many times in European football league such uncontrolled situation has existed. The discipline of sociology develops the collective sense of discipline and social control. Crucial matches or tournament require this collective sense of discipline and social control. Therefore for a successful finishing of crucial tournaments factors under sociology like social control and self discipline is highly required.

8. Group Dynamics

More the sociological effect on team members more will be the group dynamics. To work in same team or group and putting all effort collectively to gain good performance as a team/or group require group dynamics .Sociology has given much importance on this aspect of socialization and this shows the importance of sociology in the field of physical education and sports.

9. Individual as Social Beings

Sociology helps individual to become a valuable member of a society. It enables a man to be good social being and a good social being understands the importance of social values and ethics in the field of physical education and sports.

Sociology make athletes understand what kind of behaviour is acceptable to society and what not, this helps him to become a good sports person.

10. Improves Standard of Sports

Through social factors like good character, discipline, self-control, loyalty, Nationalism, respect etc. in the field of physical education and sports standard of sports also increases. The process of socialization assists in developing good sports ethics in society. Unfair attitude, Doping cases, Negative remarks etc. unsocial behaviour reduces through socialization and this no doubt increasing the standard of sports.

11. Achievement and Performance in Sports Increases

Healthy social relations with team members and others and good cooperative behaviour build confidence and motivation in players. Group Dynamics is considered an important factor for good performance of any team. Team cannot neglect the importance of social values for good performance and achievements. Sociological aspects plays important role in gaining high performance by any team or group.

12. Interdependence of Sociology and Physical Education or Sports

Physical Education and sports more strengthen the social values learned under sociology. Sports give more practical experience to the process of socialization. In physical Education and sports one get enough opportunities to implement and understand social values learned under sociology Physical Education and sports no doubt enhances the process of socialization.

13. Sociology of Sports

Sociology of sports is an area of sociology that informs us about influences of physical Education and sports on society. Therefore sociology also explains the impact of sport participation on the life of a person or society as a whole. Importance of sociology itself exists when we remind the statement "Sports is a social phenomenon"

LEADERSHIP AND GROUP DYNAMICS

A leader have magnet in heart and compass in head.

LEADERSHIP

"Leadership is the ability to score desirable actions from a group of followers voluntarily without the use of coercion."

— Alfordand Beaty

"Leadership is the activity of influencing people to strive willingly for group objectives".

— George Terry

Leadership is a dynamic ability of influencing group ion a particular situation for obtaining group objectives. It is an art, a science of enabling follow men to proceed together for the desired purpose. Leadership is a personal quality.

GROUP DYNAMICS

Every individual have a different perception, different feelings, different capability and different performance level but when working in a group these dynamic processes needed to be adopted so that predefined goal can be achieved in a collective manner is group dynamics.

Group dynamics is the adjustment within the team and this leads to better performance. Group dynamics and sports performance is directly proportional to each other. Better the Group dynamics better the performance of that group will be.

LEADERSHIP QUALITIES

Following are some of the qualities needed in a leader:-

1. PERSONALITY

Fine personality includes good physical fitness and mental alertness.

2. LOYALTY

Loyalty is the highly needed quality in any leader. Good citizenship and patriotism is resulted due to loyalty.

3. SINCERITY

Leader must be sincere enough towards the responsibility.

4. COOPERATIVE AND COORDINATIVE

Qualities of good cooperation and coordinative abilities are desirable in leader.

5. DISCIPLINE OR DUTIFULNESS

For effective leadership discipline dutifulness is essentially required for making productive effort by a leader.

6. PATIENCE

With patience good self control or calmly performing/ working increases the performance and help to proceed for better output.

7. IMPARTIALITY

Unbiased decisions, unfavourable behaviour is essentially needed in any leader to work effectively with group.

8. TACTFULNESS INTELLIGENCY INDUSTRIOUSNESS

Leader must have the tactics to make everyone validly happy and the skills to overcome hurdles tactfully, intelligently with a creative effort.

9. RELIABLE THINKING OR REALISTIC

Reliable thinking or realistic approach motivates leaders to choose the right and acceptable ways to move ahead as a team for achieving goal.

10. ENGAGING PERSONALITY AND ENDURANCE (WORK POWER)

A desire to learn more and always involved himself for one or the other require work is desirable in any leader. This is actually the quality of working ability and good utilization of leisure time.

11. MOTOR ABILITIES AND PHYSICAL SKILLS

Good Motor capacity and physical skills makes leadership more influencing. Physical Education need these abilities mainly for displaying good demonstrations to groups.

12. PUBLIC RELATIONS

Development of any kind is impossible in isolation. Leaders must always be in good and friendly public relations. Recognition, influence on others is only gained if one has good and wide public relations.

There are number of leadership qualities need in a leader. In short the word 'LEADER' itself assists us in remembering those qualities.

L - Loving nature loyalty

E - Enthusiasm

A - Alertness, Ability to handle situational load

D - Dedicative, Dutifulness, Discipline.

E - Engaging personality

R - Reasonable thinking, Reliability

S - Sincerity, Self control, Social ability

H - Hard-working, Honesty

I - Industriousness, Interest in related work/task

P - Personality, Physical skills

DEVELOPMENT OF LEADERSHIP QUALITIES AND GROUP DYNAMICS

Physical Education provides large scope to develop leadership qualities and group dynamics through its various means. Following points describes the ways through which the leadership qualities and group dynamics are developed.

1. GAMES AND SPORTS

Games and sports develop those qualities practically which are needed in social life. It teaches leaders to work under rules, work together to score goal. Sacrifice ball to give good pass etc. Therefore its no doubt that 'Games and Sports' provide lots of opportunities to experience various types of situations to deal with, opportunities to work collectively in a systematic manner, opportunities to correct the drawbacks and work on those drawbacks etc. which ultimately helps in producing good leaders.

Games are sports are thus one of the best means of developing leadership qualities and group dynamics which any individual happily accepts or adopts.

2. KNOWLEDGE

Providing good knowledge bring lot of confidence and awareness in students. A child with good and latest knowledge helps in developing desired qualities to become influencing leader. The best method to develop leadership qualities is to providing relates and latest knowledge with feeding could interest in students.

3. PLANNING ABILITIES

Systematic planning is the quality required in every leader. Teaching the importance of systematic planning and that too well in advance is very beneficial for development of good leaders. In physical Education planning of strategies and planning of training programmes teaches individuals the importance of planning. Good planning abilities naturally assist individuals to become good leaders.

4. CONFIDENCE LEVEL

The more confident, the better leader one is. Good confidence level is highly needed in every leader. Physical Education through its various types of activities like lead up games, mass demonstrations, marching and drills etc. create good confidence level within the child. Increased physical fitness through various physical activities develops confidence in students which also assists in producing good and effective leaders.

5. PROVIDING MOTIVATION

Physical Education Programmes designed to motivate the participants. Individuals must be motivated to become good leaders. If students are properly motivated they will get more interest to become leaders. Developing motivation in children's helps in developing leadership qualities.

6. ANALIZATION AND EVALUATION

Analization or Evaluation educational learning by

teachers or by self is essential to realize what more is needed to improve one. Analizing the performance level presents the drawbacks also, therefore to workout for improvement it is essential that drawbacks must be known. Regular analization and evaluation of students is needed to develop lacking qualities of leadership.

7. COLLECTIVE EFFORT

Any task performed with collective effort develops the understanding, responsibilities in the group members. Physical Educational activities like mass displays assist in development of up given qualities which is essential for leaders. Therefore collective effort develops leadership qualities.

PHYSICAL EDUCATION (GAMES AND SPORTS) AS MAN'S CULTURAL HERITAGE

Culture is a belief, a practice, a custom, which has its root in the past and has been transmitted from the past generation to their succeeding generation. Each nation having its own values or practices and as these valves or practices are accepted by the new generation, it becomes their cultural heritage, i.e. YOGA, it was practiced by our ancestors and they perform it as a sacred workout. Slowly it becomes tradition in Indian culture. Now a days Yoga is a popular sport also and we having competitions in Yoga at various levels. This strengthens the belief that Games and sports is our cultural Heritage.

Several games now familiar across the world are their origin as culture of one or the other society (nation). ARCHERY was well-accepted culture of many Nations in Ancient time, which has now existed as very popular and competent sport. In India chess, playing cards, Gully Danda, Kabbadi etc. were very existing as modified sports and games.

Even if we talk about basic human activities like walking, running, jumping, throwing etc. were as essential to human beings in ancient time as these are now a days. All such kind of survival activities become part of our culture dances like Bharatanatyam, Bhangra, Kathak, Katha Kali, Kuchipudi etc. show Indian culture and on the side they are good physical activities as well.

Games and sports are correctly considered as very valuable culture of any nation and it must be treated and enhanced as cultural heritage. Following points clears us more about the statement "Games and Sports as man's cultural Heritage"

1. Being passed on generation to generation

Games and sports are rich cultural heritage of every nation, which is being accepted by next generation. Like other culture Games and sports is also a practice or a tradition which has its root in the past and has been transmitted from the past generation to their succeeding generation. Gradually the ancient physical activities existed in a modified manner, as our other culture is also modified. Games and sports has its valves since time immemorial and human beings had grownup in sports culture and this culture is an important heritage of every country.

2. Culture itself as games/Sports

Many classical Indian dances, which are part of our valuable culture since long back, are also good physical activities. Archery Disc throw, racing wrestling etc. comes under ancient culture but these are popular sports also. Gladiatorial Combats in Rome Olympic in Athens Lingiads in Sweden is an important cultural heritage of respective countries but these comes under games and sports as well. Therefore games and sports is also an important cultural heritage.

3. Importance of culture shown in sports

Sports and Games were integral part of many societies and many sports societies and many sports were as culture in many nations. Because of ancient Olympics is culture in Athens, the people there were good sports persons or sports being. In every age we could analyze the influence of culture on sports. Ancient Greeks then consisted of numerous small states, was of very belligerent attitudes and this behaviour existed in their sports activities and tough physical training. Organization of sports athletic events wrestling, racings, throwing etc. by various nations in national festivals shows sports and games as culture. Culture of sports in ancient Greece was always in priority and Truce was observed inspite of their belligerent attitude during the Olympics. It indicate us the moral importance of this cultural heritage.

4. Exchange of culture by sports

There are many such activities like Archery, Wrestling, Throwing, Chess Racing, Martial Arts, Yoga etc. which indicated culture of many societies and at present these activities are well recognized as popular sports. Many Indian cultural programmes (like Yoga Bhangra, kathak) are beneficial physical activities. It is some times therefore hard to differentiate between culture and sports.

5. Modification of Culture

A game named CHATURANG was an important part of ancient Indian culture, now known as CHESS is the modification of culture. Sports and Games were integral part of every nation's culture and modification is the requirement. But this modification doesn't changes the culture. The sports like chess, archery, wrestling, and racings etc. were an important part of culture in past also and will remain an important part in future also.

GAMES AND SPORTS AS MAIN CULTURAL HERITAGE

It is no doubt that "Games and sports" is cultural heritage of every nation. Since from ancient time human being is well involved in physical activities in one or the other form.

Hunting was activity for survival of primitive man, later existed as famous sport of Javelin, shooting etc. the best way to prove given statement "Games and sports an man's cultural heritage is going to Historical Background of physical activities in different nations.

1. GREECE- Greece has contributed a lot in making games and sports as cultural heritage. Greece was the first nation who adopted sports competitions as National Festivals. History of Greece (in Games and sports mainly) can be divided in four sports-

i. Homeric period.

ii. Spartan period

iii. Early Athenian period

iv. Later Athenian period.

i. Homeric period. This period has recorded early Grecian life, where a great interest of people is found towards physical activities like wrestling, shooting, chariot Races, gymnastics. Other cultural activities like dancing, arts were also famous needed physical involvements.

ii. Spartan period. Spartans were basically strict followers of military regulations. They are recognized as Man of action. Touch physical activities was the regular programme for every individual. Every effort was made to keep them physically fit. Wrestling, jumping, throwing were their famous sports. Spartan had introduced Ball games also.

iii. Early Athenian Period- Early Athenian were democratic in nature but they never underestimated military abilities. Here also tough physical activities were essential part of educational curriculum. They were famous for celebrating mainly four national athletic contests (Pannellenic games).

a) Olympic- In honour of God Zeus celebrated every first year of Olympiad.

b) Pythian games- in honour of God Apollo. Celebrated every 3rd year of Olympiad.

c) Isthmian games- In honour of God of sea, celebrated every 2nd and 4th year of Olympiad.

d) Neemean games- In honour of God Zeus celebrated every 2nd years of Olympiad.

iv. Later Athenian period- this period generally known as Golden period. By this period sports existed as profession also. Apart from physical activities, other concerning activities related with fitness and health became; popular like medical Gymnastics, corrective exercises.

Rome- In early Rome physical activities used for improving skills of war, getting courage. Dance was an integral event of their cultural programme. Combat sports like wrestling, sword fighting were very famous earlier but then existed the brutal gladiatorial combats 264 BC. Chariot races, throwing events and minor children recreational games were also on demand. Gambling was also very famous in Roman society. Thermac (thermal Bath-rooms) was in good utilization for recreation or relaxation.

Germany- Germany has contribute a lot in making games and sports as world's cultural heritage by giving new concepts in physical activities.

Johan -B. Basedow (1713-1790) who is recognized as founder of modern physical.Education pvt. Every effort to popularize physical activities in schools.

Johann Guts Muths (1959-1839) who is regarded as father of German gymnastics introduced gymnastics in schools and popularized other like swimming, wrestling, balance exercises, hiking as part of physical Educational programme. Guts Muths also introduces Recreational activities for better development of personality.

Activities like Football, gymnastics, swimming, indoor games are extremely popular in Germany.

Japan

Physical activities mainly defensive art exists clearly within the culture of Japan. Fencing, Japanese wrestling, archery, obscuring hunting are very cultural and exists since ancient time. Budo (Military art) was very religious also since 1880 when Professor Jigard Kend who invented Judo many traditional schools are teaching this defensive activity has become part of their culture.

Sweden

Gymnastics, Fencing, Swimming are regarded as

their traditional activities. Medical gymnastics (exercises for good body posture) is also famous. Weather conditions do not favour outdoor games much but winter sports like skating are popular since long back. Indoor games are therefore more close to people here. In Sweden 'Lingiad' named after 'per Henrik Ling' is celebrated as sports festival.

Denmark

Denmark is the first European country to make games and sports or physical activities as essential programme in school curriculum. Rifle club was formed to teach shooting and military drills in Denmark . Traditional Danis gymnastic (Rhythmic exercises) has become world famous.

USA

Sports and games is in culture of U.S.A. since ancient time. With little modification and need of people many games like Basket ball (1892), Volley Ball (1892), American Foot ball, Baseball, Handball, Rugby, Golf introduced in U.S.A. Track field and gymnastic is also very popular. Combat sports (Wrestling, boxing etc.) is in demand always. Physical education is compulsory subject in schools in America.

India

Games and sports in ancient India since Vedic age (2000-1000 B.C.) is regarded as very prestigious and royal activity. Archery, horse riding, chariot racing, gambling were very popular activities slowly passed on to whole world. Yoga (Yug) is traditional activity in India performed by every one. In Epic age Gurukuls Physical activity was performed regularly. Indian warriors were specialized in Archery, wrestling, sword fighting, disc throwing Javelin throwing etc. Kho Kho, Kabaddi etc., are very famous and regarded as indigenous games. Folk dance of every state involves lot of physical workout. India has also introduced many Rhythmic exercises and mass display like BHARTIUM. World famous game of Badminton is discovered in India. Cricket, Soccer, Volley ball, Basket ball are other famous games.

SOCIOLOGICAL APPROACH AND VALUE EDUCATION THROUGH PHYSICAL EDUCATION PROGRAMME

If the aim of Education is enrichment of personality, Physical Education contributes to much extent. If the aim of Education is self/ realization, again no doubt physical Education provides opportunities to develop the sense of self/ realization. To achieve every philosophical realization aim and objective of Education, physical, Education play an important role and assist in developing those objectives more practically. Therefore, it is said that physical education is an integral part of total education process.

Whole Educational process become more easy and efficient when physical Education put its contributions physical education is an essential part of total education process. Secondary Education Commission (1952-53) enlisted four aims of education i.e.

(i) Development of democratic approach,

(ii) Improvement of vocational efficiency,

(iii) Development of personality and

(iv) Development of qualities of leadership.

Physical education puts its great contribution in developing these qualities in an individual.

Two statements 'A sound mind lies in a sound body'

and 'physical Education an integral part of total Education' is one statement empowers the other statement. A complete personality is consisted of healthy body and healthy mind. In other words it can be said physical educations assist whole educational process in developing all round personality. Only theoretical approach may produce a sound mind, but for a sound body physical approach is required. Therefore only class room education itself cannot be considered as a complete educational programme until and unless physical education is regarded as an integral part of the programme. Relationship of physical education with general education is well recognized and understood. It is therefore, physical education found essentially place in regular curriculum of every education institution.

Following given points present, the assistance of physical education in valuing education.

1. Interesting- sports and games, recreation and other physical activities create interest in students and they become motivated to follow educational programmes. Physical Education makes education programme more interesting. Physical education is a source recreation, relaxation; keep students happy and enjoyable, which make students energetic and interesting in the total educational programmes.

2. Effective and easy learning

Only classroom learning in an educational programme may not be much effective. Learning of social valves like cooperation, adjustment, teamwork, self-control etc. is more effective and practical in physical education. Student's participation in different physical activities provides ample opportunities to learn many educational valves. Therefore physical education assist total education programme in effective and easy learning of students.

3. Healthy approach

Physical education develops competitive spirit with a cooperative attitude. This aspect bring programme in the total education programme. Students try to perform their best in classrooms or in Examinations with a cooperative attitude. Apart from this, physical activities make students physical fit and mentally healthy. This can be concluded as physical education makes total education programme a healthy approach.

4. Responsibilities and Discipline

Physical Education through its various activities assists in developing sense of responsibility and discipline in students. These qualities make possible the smooth and effective running of education programmes. Therefore, total education programme possibly achieve the motive of producing valuable citizens for the country.

5. Knowledge

Physical education coves wide range of subjects like Physiology, human anatomy, psychology, sport medicine, health education etc., which involve huge knowledge for the students. Learning of healthy education first aid, communicable diseases, diet and nutrition like topics is very essential for children's and adolescents. Updating of knowledge is one of the main objectives of any education programme. Physical Education contributes a lot also in relation to providing beneficial knowledge to students.

6. Growth and Development

During the phases of infant to adolescent individual requires special attention for their proper growth and development. Absence of any physical activities may harm the normal growth and development. In this stage students require some specific kind of physical activities, which assist in their growth and development. Education curriculum must be involve such activities for proper growth and development of students.

7. Friendship and Relationship

Sports and other physical activities provide an environment for every one to feel enjoyable and understand each other. Physical education assist in strength ring relationships and develop the quality of group dynamics it improves student - student and student - teacher relationship Good relations bring progress in the total education programme.

8. Other

Physical education develops many other such qualities behaviour or attitude that make physical education an important part of total education programme. Physical education develops leadership qualities, and personal habits acceptable attitude. Creativeness in students.

Physical education therefore plays an important role in putting the value education.

MEANING AND FUNCTIONS OF FAMILY AND ITS IMPORTANCE AS A SOCIAL INSTITUTION

INTRODUCTION- (FAMILY AS SOCIAL INSTITUTION)

"Social institution is a structure of society that is organized to meet the needs of people through well established procedures."

—Sir Bogardus.

Family is one of the most important institution of the society and having direct influence on the related individual or group. Social institution here is referred as an organization which works with collective effort to gain some specific purpose. Social institutions are actually representing some set of individuals within the society with specific objectives, club or Team or family or Government etc. can be placed as example. Every social institution works with some definite rules and regulations though some rules are some times not followed by individuals. Framed with common assents like in a non-vegetarian family

Each member may agree to this rule. In the other side it may the case that one member desire to eat non-vegetable food. Therefore some times rules not compulsorily followed by individual member or more members. It is also to be cleared that some rules of any social institution must be compulsorily followed or obeyed by every member.

Such rules lays down the modes of conduct expected and if not obeyed by members of that social institution warning or punishment is given. Therefore the social institutions like.

- Family
- Education Institution.
- Friends circle.
- State etc. moulds.

"Family is a social grouping of members which are united by bonds of kinship".

"Family is a miniature social organization including at least two generation and characteristically formed upon the blood bond relation".

— Summer and Keller

"Family is a group defined by saw relationship sufficiently precise and endorsing to provide for the procreation and up bringing of children"

— MacIver. F

"Family is a system of relationship between parents and children".

— Clarke

"A family is a group of persons united by the ties of marriage, blood or adoption constituting a single. Household , interacting and inter communicating with each other in their respective social role of husband and wife, mother and father , son and daughter brother and sister, and creating and maintaining a common culture".

—Burgessand Locke

"Family is a group defined by sex relationship sufficiently precise and endorsing to provide for the procreation and upbringing of children".

— MacIver & Page

Family is a group of persons who live under the same roof and are connected by nuclear and kinship ties and own a consciousness of kind on the basis of locality, interest and mutuality of an obligation.

"Family is the centre of love and affection, best place for education and the first placer for the child".

— Pestalozei

"Family is an informal educational centre where the learning is provided by Mother-father, brothers and sisters or the individuals having blood relation or marriage relation".

"Family is a biological social unit composed of a husband, wife and their children"

— Eziot and Merizz

"In a family mother is the true nurse and father is the true teacher of a child".

— Pausseau

"Family is a group of persons whose relations to one another are based upon contranguinity and who are therefore kind to another".

— Davis

MEANING OF FAMILY

The word "FAMILY" is derived from the Roman word "Famulus" which means attendant or servant. 'Attendant' or 'servant' here refers to individuals willingly serve the persons related by blood or marriage.

Family is a primary social group consisting of a mother, father, brothers and sisters. The child continues to identify himself with the family throughout the life period and thus family is the only social institution which exists always. Family is said to be the oldest and the most important informal active agency of education. The child gets the first social environment from the family from which the child fulfils his physical, mental, cultural needs. Family is also the most influential group/social institution and plays key role in the total process of socialization. In some texts family is also referred as "HOME" the basis of the statement that family is considered as group of people sharing a home. Family is the union of husband and wife or the individuals residing together which may include from mother, father, their children to aunts uncles, cousins etc. Family is a primary unit/group of interacting personalities in which each personality has its definite role and responsibility. The Indian society is formalistic in nature and primarily provides social recognition. Family satisfies the related members in many respects and influences the growth/ development of a child. Family plays an important and continues role in the education of the child. Family is a miniature social group which forms the basis of social processes. It is a socialized group of closely related individuals which exhibit standards of behaviour. Family is an important source of adjustment in whole society. In family child gets its first lessons in love, cooperation, social values etc., from the family members like mother, father. Growth of a child is influenced by the environment presenting in the related family. Acquisition of habits by children is an example of it. Family is treated as the first learning institution of an individual and it is rightly said that as is the family, so will be the society. Family having its influences in society and therefore the importance of this primary group can never be under estimated in the socialization process.

Nuclear Family-Nuclear family can be described as a family comprising of a mother, a father and their children,. Nuclear family is characterized with single Home in which mother and father live with their dependent children. In the modern society nuclear families are existing more and mainly found in cities.

Nuclear families are mainly supported by one or two earning hands and the domestic budget scale is not big enough generally as compared to joint families.

JOINT FAMILIES - Joint families can be described as a big family where generations are living together this includes mother, father with their married children and their kids. Joint family is characterized with single home and extended family. In villages joint families still exists with good family spirit. In a joint family the members by relation are parents, their married children, grand children, which also give birth to relation like uncles, aunts, cousins. Joint families are supported by number of earning hands and the domestic budget scale is by enough generally if compared with nuclear families.

FUNCTIONS/IMPORTANCE OF FAMILY AS SOCIAL INSTITUTION

The assistance and guidance given by family to its members for proper growth and development with the society are the functions performed by the family. The functions of family are also explained as importance of families in society. Following are the functions/ importance of family.

1. PHYSICAL AND HEALTH DEVELOPMENT-

One of the most important functions of family is assist in gaining good physique and healthy body. Creating and maintaining of favourable opportunity by the family for effective physical and health development of children is an essential function of any family. The physical and health development of any family member depends on many factors like family habits, balanced diet, wearing tradition, exercise schedule, sleep work load, medical assistance family and personal hygiene etc. Therefore the effectiveness of any family of performing these aspects well decides the physical and health development of its members.

2. BIOLOGICAL FUNCTIONS

Reproduction is considered as the main function of any family. Reproduction of next generation is that function of family which carries the social process of family inheritance forward. Biological function is the most responsible function of any family therefore must be given every thought before undergoing this function efficiently and social values must also be taken into consideration.

3. INTELLECTUAL DEVELOPMENT

Proper mental development of child is the another important function of family. Family provide rich intellectual environment to child which increase his mental abilities, intelligence, quick thinking, effective reasoning, which ultimately promote the society. Acquisition of healthy habits, creative nature and productive interests is done through the intellectual development function of family. This function plays an important role in the development of any child. Intellectual development is the basis of further development and promotions in healthy living.

4. EMOTIONAL DEVELOPMENT

Process of bringing emotional stability in child is an equally essential function of family as others. This function includes the aspects like love, affection, anger, competition, cooperation etc., which must be controlled efficiently. Proper care and guidance of children by parents (family) develop the emotional status. Emotional stability is required to play effective role in society controlling of emotions in children highly depends upon the family atmosphere.

5. CHARACTER DEVELOPMENT

Family lays the foundation of character. Good moral character of a child increases the family status. Family is highly responsible in the development of character of related member. This function includes the aspects like honesty, ethics, responsibilities, truthfulness, faithfulness, regards, sympathy, sincerity etc. Disruptive behaviour of parents may lead to undemanding behaviour of children also. Parents in the family should take every care of child for this proper character development.

6. EDUCATIONAL FUNCTION

Family is the fist educational institution for any child. The basic learning function starts from family. Apart from the continues learning in family, the further study of child depends on family. Parent's willingness matters a lot in this concern. It is the responsibility of every family to perform this function efficiently, providing education to family members is proved beneficial for whole family and the society as well.

7. ECONOMICS FUNCTION

Another important function of family is assisting teaching the child in understanding the economic demands of every individual. Important function of providing vocational or professional training to children is highly required. By performing this function family make children self dependent or standing on their own feet. This function includes the characteristics like efficient working, proper utilization of resources, balanced budget/expenditure etc., which also lead to develop society.

8. SOCIAL DEVELOPMENT

Child learns or develops social values in the family. Family plays an important role in the total social process. Social development first takes place in a family and this function mainly includes aspects like cooperation, understanding, common thought, wellness, mutual relations, togetherness, belongingness etc. This function is the basis of socialization and accomplished of recognition or understanding of social values. Family realizes child the importance of society and necessity of co-existence with the society.

9. CIVIC FUNCTION

Another important responsibility on family is to produce a good sense of citizenship in child. This valuable function of the family is essentially performed for the better development of nation/society as a whole. This function includes characteristics like responsibility, obedience, faithfulness, tolerance, discipline, patriotism. Family assist in realizing learning and discharging duties/responsibilities to the child.

10. PSYCHOLOGICAL FUNCTION

Family provide effective psychological satisfaction to its members/children. Family performs the psychological function by providing mental satisfaction, relaxation, assist in overcoming anxiousness confident, overcoming stress, etc. Healthy psychology of an individual leads to healthful living procedures. Psychological development of any child also depends on the mental attitude of family members.

11. CULTURAL FUNCTION

Cultural heritage of any family is a valuable thing of

every family. Function of transmitting these cultural heritage tō its children is very recognized and auspicious function performed by the family. This function of family helps in saving the historic culture and tradition of one family rather the society. The cultural function includes customs, social/family values, conventions, traditions which make our society more developed and united and unique.

12. COLLECTIVE EFFORT

Family members work collectively for some common objective. This function of collective effort performed by family brings progression and development is the family. Child learns cooperative qualities through the function of collective effort. Acquisition of this function/quality by individuals/child provide favourable atmosphere for the society to achieve high goals and develop faster.

13. RELIGIOUS FUNCTION

A child gain religious knowledge and values from the family. The religious development in any child is brought by its family. Performance of this function by family makes children living more meaningful, interesting and active. This function in general may also include daily worship of respected God. This function helps in developing the quality of showing devotion to God and every religion. Society is highly influential and benefited by practising religious functions by family.

14. SHELTER AND SECURITY

Child is provided shelter and security by the family. The function of shelter and security is one of the basic requirements of every human being. Family works for the development of child. Providing of shelter and security helps in this task. This function of protection/

support assist child to learn effectively and develop confidently. In all the stages of life child/member expects from the family as a whole to perform this function. In the childhood, adolescent and old age the function of shelter and security is performed will every care by the family.

15. EXPERIENCES

All the initial experiences of life is learned by the child from family. The experience from walking to talking,, behavioural experiences, dealing with situations, overcoming problems, cooperation, togetherness etc., provided by the family time to time. It is the usefulness of this function of the family that child/member learns the processes of development and empower himself. Human beings gets new experiences in every walk of life and the past leant experiences assist him to understand the new experience.

16. HABIT FORMING FUNCTION

Family plays important role in realizing, creating, good habits and maintaining those habits by the child for the welfare of mankind. Development of productive habits in the child is beneficial for the society/nation. Family makes children understanding the differences in good and bad habits and then put its effort for the adaptation of good habits by the child.

17. RECREATIONAL FUNCTION

Family chooses some activities to get engaged in a constructive manner during leisure time. This function refreshes the family members and the enjoyment or satisfactions they get make them more energetic and productive. The voluntary participation of family members reduces their tensions, tiredness and they become fresher to perform their daily respective tasks perfectly. This function is therefore having great importance for the development of family and society as a whole. Recreational function helps in developing leisure skills and interests in family members.

18. CARETAKING FUNCTION

Family plays efficiently a role of caretaker of child. Family takes every care of child and provide suitable atmosphere for development. Making available necessary items. Proper diet, confident and psychological balanced and secured life are the main aspects under this function of family. This function helps children for their growth and development and this also increases their standard of living.

4

BIOLOGICAL FOUNDATION OF PHYSICAL EDUCATION

Concepts of Nature and Nurture

It has been customary for a long time to regard nature and nurture as mutually antagonistic and exclusive factors that determine the behaviour of individuals. The inheritance of traits and the effect of environment have provided the battleground for long and heated arguments. With the advance of genetics as a science of inheritance, the exclusive character of one influence or the other has been seriously challenged. Long accustomed to authoritarian views about nature, modern man retains in his beliefs, customs and speech notions about nature of an exceedingly bizarre character. These range from the doctrine of man's inheritance evil nature to the concept that nature is always right.

The study of genetics has afforded the basis for new interpretations of nature. The failures of man to build a good world are due neither to his inheritance evilness nor to his slavish devotion to and following of nature. On the contrary, the present incapacity to utilize constructively the forces of the environment and his own potential powers forms the problem.

Society rapidly changing under the force of man's invention, must now face the problem of human behaviour. Thus, the crucial tasks we confront in physical education are those of nurture rather than nature. We are learning slowly, but surely that to get a better world to live in, we must secure better living in the world rather than attempt to secure a transformation of nature.

The rejection of the idea that nature exerts an all-pervading influence in human life does not deny to nature a position of considerable importance. This influence, however, often relates to an earlier life of man. Man is still equipped by nature to live in an environment vastly different from the life that now is, as a result of science, art, reasoning, habit, language, tools, books, and various customs of his race. Hence, each new individual must unlearn much of his nature in order to live with others in the crowded co-ordinated life of industrial society.

By nature man cries from pain and fights for things he wants, he grabs and snatches from others. By nurture of particular kinds, he learns to merit what he takes, and to earn or deserve the satisfaction of his wants. The present understanding of nature rejects the notion that nature is always right or always wrong or half and half. It recognizes that the individual possess drives, urges and impulses to certain kinds of behaviour and that these should be strengthened at times, weakened at times, and completely checked at times.

Physical education in the selection of activities should recognize that man is prepared by nature to engage in certain kinds of activity. Many of the persistent problems in physical education today are clarified by reference to the facts of nature. The fact that man presents in the racial patterns of his nervous system certain underlying predispositions to function in well-defined motor activities characterized in type and quality by his motor experiences over thousands of years, that he is urged on by his very nature to exploit these established organizations, and that, under proper guidance, such expressions may be made to serve high causes and noble ends is of outstanding import.

Nature proclivities of man represent enormous changes from original traits. Learning and nurture in its various forms are represented in the liking of boys for fishing, sport and adventure since nature knows nothing of sport records. Nature's tendencies may go as far as to enjoy throwing a small object and swinging a club like thing, but the majority of the sports of youth are modifications and adaptation of these early proclivities. Such modifications are natural activities in their basic patterns, but all reflect the influence of nurture.

Today, biological and cultural evolutions have far reaching implications. In ancient days, it was required for the existence of man to indulge in various kinds of physical activities. Now, it is necessary for human beings to keep them fit to sustain their biological posture proper. Physical activities are practised to keep an individual emotionally and mentally fit. An inheritance of structure and function has been brought by biological evolution which has aroused requirement of care and attention. Modern age is age of technology and this kind of living has affected to physiques of general people to a lot of extent. Not only this, they have brought various negative effect on the mental abilities of people. One should remember that a sound mind can only reside in a sound body.

Meanings of Growth and Development

Generally word growth and development are used

synonymously, however, there is a difference in the meanings of these concepts. Technically, growth of an individual means increase in mass, while development is the organization of that tissue into functional units or powers. Development of the child can be judged in part by growth, but growth may occur without a corresponding development.

Nutrition and various hygienic factors condition growth and development. While physical education influences growth, its chief interest is in development.

Growth

The process through which body increases in size and shape is known as growth. Process of growth is biological in nature. An increase in mass is termed as growth. From the first growth of the fertilized ovum until maturity of the individual is reached numerous forces determine growth. Some organs evens continue to grow in old age also. Thus, a quantitative increase in the size and shape of the body is termed as growth. When these organs changes in size and shape, it is known as physical growth. All the organs of body grow at different rate. For this reason, growth is considered a tangible biological process. In this process, various organs of the human body develop in respect of size, height and weight. There occurs an increase in the size of cells of body and muscles. In body structure, various kinds of changes take place and these changes are of quantitative nature.

Development

A process which brings human body towards the point of maturity is known development. In other words, process of development is concerned with advancement of human body. The various kinds of qualitative changes that takes place in human body are considered development in true sense.

Process of development is more concerned with external factors. If all these external factors are not ensured properly, development will not take place properly. It can be said that the process under which capabilities of an individual get expanded which provide him with greater facility in functioning is known as development.

Although concepts of development and growth are different, but they are inter-related to each other. Growth is a means to achieve development. For the development of functional capacities of human beings, growth functions as a basis. At no stage, it is possible to acquire proper development with improper growth. Development of an individual is concerned with his mental, intellectual and social aspects. Development process consists of acquisition of skills and knowledge of various fields.

Thus it can be said that both the processes of growth and development are complimentary to each other and it is not possible to achieve one successfully without achieving another. Development is a life long procedure while growth is a limited period process. An human being grow upto a certain age or period in his life but process of development continues throughout the lifetime.

Learning

When an individual acquires knowledge of some skill, he is said to have learnt that skill. Learning can be of different kinds and every kind of learning brings about a kind of change in the behaviour of individuals.

With the process of growth, a child's body becomes more heavier and taller. With the result of development, capacities of human body increases and organs of body become more capable to understand various kinds of complex functions. As an individual becomes maturer, his systems become more adapted to handle various kinds of situations. As a result of an individual's interaction with the environment, he continues to learn. All these processes are not fully independent in nature, but they are inter-related to each other in one way and other.

Maturation

Maturation is a physiological development that occur in human body from time to time. This kind of development is qualitative in nature. This process occurs as a result of biological functions.

In development of a child, various processes play important roles. These processes are growth, maturation and learning. These are related to each other and function properly in association with each other.

Kinds of Development

As development is a life long process, it can be in different forms. There are three kinds of developments which take place in an individual, which are :—

a. Social Development,

b. Motor Development,

c. Mental Development.

Social Development : The process which helps in developing the qualities of human behaviour is known as social development. These qualities include quality of working in co-operation and co-ordiation with others and quality to lead other persons.

Motor Development : Development of general body control, fine motor skills and large muscle movements are considered part of this kind of development. Such developments take place with the help of movements like running, jumping and throwing.

Mental Development : With the increase in age, mental abilities of an individual also increases. Such type of increase in mental capabilities of human beings is known as mental development. With such kind of development, an individual becomes able to distinguish between different kind of things, learning difficult skills or things, and gets reasoning ability.

Thus on the basis of above discuss it can be said that there lies a difference between growth and development. The points of differences that exist between these concepts are as follows :—

a. One can see the process of growth in an individual, however, it is not possible to see the process of development.

b. It is possible to measure growth in physical terms, but it is not possible to measure development in such terms.

c. Growth is such a process which lasts only for a limited time. After a certain age, process of growth ceases to take place, however, development is a long process, which lasts throughout the life time. Right from the time a child takes birth in the world upto the time he dies, process of development goes on.

d. Heredity of an individual plays an important role in defining the limits of growth, while external factors affect process of development to a lot of extent.

Fundamental Principles of Growth and Development

Both the processes of growth and development are guided by certain fundamental principles. These principles should be kept in mind while formulating the physical education programmes. Some of the important principles of growth and development are as follows :—

a. It is with the interaction of heredity and environment that processes of growth and development take place.

b. A specific genetic sequence is being followed by processes by growth and development. The nature of these processes do not remain same at different stages. They become complex from simple state with span of time.

c. Process of growth and development are long term procedures. They are gradual in nature. These are co-related with the life span of an individual. Long the life span of an individual, long will be these processes.

d. Growth and development processes are creative in nature. As a result of these processes, various kinds of changes take place in functional and behavioural features of the individual.

e. Quality of germs and other external factors affect these processes to a lot of extent.

f. Rate of increase of both these processes varies from each other. In each individual, these processes take place with different pace.

Factors that Affect Processes of Growth and Development

Processes of growth and development can be affected by various factors, some of which are : Environmental

Factors, Genetic Factors, Nutritional Factors and Physical Education Programmes.

All these factors affect growth and development in different manners, which has been discussed in the following manner :—

Effect of Environmental Factors on Growth and Development

It is firstly very necessary to understand what factors are included in the specific category of environmental factors. Factors like healthy traditions, geographical conditions, education, health related facilities, and social codes are some of the important components of this category.

Effect of Genetic Factors on Growth and Development

That branch of biology which deals with the heredity is known as Genetics. In all the human bodies, some genes are present which help in passing some characteristics of parents to the children. Patterns of growth from one generation to another are being controlled by genes, because of which they are considered the most powerful of living forces. The fundamental traits which are being transferred from parents to children are height, speed, agility etc. If the genes of the parents are weak, then child can be affected by various diseases or some diseases which parents faces, can be faced by their children also.

Effect of Nutritional Factors on Growth and Development

To its optimum limits, well balanced diet, climatic conditions and stages of growth and development affect pace of the processes of growth and development to a lot of extent.

Effect of Physical Education Programme on Growth and Development

While designing the physical education programme for school and college children, their needs and requirements should be kept in mind. If their needs will be ignored while designing such programme, no positive results can be obtained, otherwise, possibilities of getting negative results will arise.

It is believed by experts that all the teachers or physical educators should have thorough knowledge of each and every aspect relating to growth and development. Now the question arises that why it is necessary for all the teachers to have such knowledge. A teacher imparts knowledge to a large number of students and these students differ from each other in various respects. All they belong to different socio-economic backgrounds, environments, caste and have different genders. Because of difference in all these factors, there arises a lot of difference between all the children. In their level of education, these factors play an important role.

The basic aim of each and every teacher is to impart education to students. It is well known that there are some qualities already present in all the students, which are being explored by teacher in such a way that students can learn the things easily. No teacher can exploit such qualities unless and until he has thorough knowledge about the qualities different students possess. It is very necessary for him to have a thorough knowledge of fundamental principles of growth and development. As a student passes through different age groups, various kinds of characteristics emerge because of all these factors. Teacher should have proper knowledge about these kind of different characteristics. He should have thorough knowledge of factors which affect the processes of growth and development.

Students are considered to be a treasure for a nation and a teacher plays an important role in bringing desirable changes in the behaviour of children. In this way, teachers create good and responsible citizens for the nation in an indirect way. They play an important role in the process of national development. Not only this, if teacher has the knowledge of various aspects of growth and development, he can without any problems, understand the students in terms of their past and can predict their future in advance.

FUNDAMENTAL FEATURES OF GROWTH AND DEVELOPMENT

From the above discussion, some of the features of growth and development become clear, which can be explained in following manner :—

a. Growth is a creative process which begins from the moment a living organism takes birth. All the anatomical structures are present in all children right from the moment of their birth, but with passage of time, different kinds of changes take place in these structures. Size of various body parts get increased and various kinds of changes take place in his physique when he comes in direct contact with outside world. Not only this, with time a lot of changes take place in behaviour pattern of children. This is the main reason that a child of five year differs from a child of fifteen years to a lot of extent. All these changes take place because of process of growth and various kinds of behavioural forms get created by this process. It is because of this process that child, who at one time could not stand independently, begins to run and even chase others. It is because of this reason it is said that growth is a creative process.

b. All living organism grow with time and to some extent it is not possible to stop process of growth. Process of growth take pace in all living organisms and one has to accept kind of changes take place in him by this process. In reality, basis of animal behaviour is nothing but process of growth. It is possible that functional capacity of child can remain undeveloped, but still process of growth will take place and bring different kinds of changes in him. Probability of getting mental growth increases in case of persons who take part in physical activities, however, process of growth does not get affected by other factors and it take place with normal pace.

c. Changed structure is the basis on which mental growth of an individual depends. A child not only grow physically but his mental capacities also develop simultaneously. If organs of perception do not develop properly, then it is found that children's level of perception and comprehension remains low. Such kind of child cannot differentiate between right and wrong things, because of which cannot take appropriate decision. With mental growth, ability of a person to accumulate experiences from the environment increases. On the basis of physical and mental developments, it is very easy to differentiate a grown-up adult and a growing child. Children do not possess very well developed muscular body because of which they cannot perform well or cannot indulge in activities requiring complex neuro-muscular co-ordination, however, it is not difficult for adults to indulge in such kinds of activities. In children, on reflex patterns, nervous system functions, however, with passage of time, reflections get conditioned and become able to produce various kinds of response patterns.

d. With growth, attitude of persons also get changed. For instance, it is found from various studies that in childhood, there is a lot of feeling of eco-centricism in children, however, with growth and maturation, this kind of attitude gets changed and take form of socio-centric. Various kinds of inner drives get arise because of instinctive urges in children and it is not possible to resist such kind of drives. Children perform only those activities by which they can get satisfaction of their self. Whenever they fail to attain their objective, they begin to react emotionally and the most obvious reaction is crying. With maturity, individual begins to understand the rules and norms of society and they begin to learn those norms. By this time, instinctive behaviours gets modified to a lot of extent and he begin to act in accordance with norms and rules of society in which he lives. Various social norms guide and direct the behaviour pattern of adults, while no knowledge of such norms is possess by children because of which sometimes they act like animals. Children perform various activities on basis of pleasure principle while adults think a lot about consequence before beginning any activity. Thus, it can be said that with growth perspective of human beings get changed and they become rational in nature.

e. Process of growth takes place when living organism gets interacted with the outside environment. Various environmental factors play an important role in determining the growth pattern of children. Processes of growth and development can take place properly only in a favourable and congenial environment. Environment in which a person lives determine the kind of relationship he will maintain with other people and kind of company he will get. Thus, these factors help to a lot of extent in adapting new skills and habits and even mould hereditary factors to a lot of extent. Process of modification will take a positive direction if environment will be of favourable nature, however, an inappropriate kind of environment will lead these process towards negative direction. One should remember that if he wants to grow a healthy and fruitful tree, then it is very necessary to provide all important constituents or things which can provide required nutritions to develop.

f. In early years of life, process of growth take place with fast pace, while this pace keeps on lowering with passage of time. When a baby is born, he seems to be very soft and tender as his body parts have very small size, but after some years, that baby turns out to be a child with comparatively hard parts and even it becomes difficult for the parents to believe that their child, who was so soft and tender at time of birth, can turn out to be of such strong physique. Various studies have been conducted to find out the pace with which process of growth take place in children and all have shown that pace of this process is more in early years of life, while with increase in age, pace of this process lowers down and after a specific age, this process stops to proceed.

g. Process of growth and development are inevitably, but limits of these processes can be set up by hereditary features. As known that various features are attained by children from his parents or other family members, which are called hereditary features. These features play an important role in defining the limits to which process of growth and development will take place. It is because of this reason that possibility of a child's height remaining low gets increased when height of his parents is also less. Thus, heredity forces play an important role in demarcating limits on processes of growth and development, however, these limits can be smashed away by various positive environmental forces.

h. Growth has various aspects, and all of them develop with different pace. It is for this reason that some children begins to toddle first while some babble first. Although generally growth pattern remains same for all children by which various experts have prescribed the standard growth pattern which should be followed by a child. If any child does not follow this pattern, then generally his parents consult any physician to find out the reason of such happening.

i. Rate of growth among children differs because of which it is said that each child grows in his own specific manner. It is because of difference in rate of growth that varied differences are seen even in twins. This fact is also responsible for producing individual differences among human beings, by which they are differentiated from each other.

j. All human beings consist of various body organs and it is not necessary that process of growth take place with same pace in all these body organs. At different times, each organ reaches its maximum dimension. However, this function takes place with a definite order. A child begins to walk after completion three months. After sometimes, marked difference can be seen in shape and width of hips. It is at the end that length of trunk and depth of chest attains peak growth speed. It is because of this reason that some children seem improportionally developed in terms of physique.

All the above features of growth and development should be kept in mind by physical educators and coaches while formulating training programme for children. By knowing growth pattern of child, great advantage can be enjoyed by sport coaches.

Growth and development are processes which take place in all human beings, but these processes have to move from various stages, which can be discussed in following manner :—

STAGES OF GROWTH AND DEVELOPMENT

All living organisms have to pass through various developmental stages. These stages of development can be defined as series of changes which an organism undergoes from embryonic stage to state of maturity. It is not easy to demarcate clear lines between various stages of development. Some experts have performed serious study on the concept that how various stages of development can be categorised and can be differentiated from each other. Reason for such kind of difficulty is that process of growth take place on a continuous base and it becomes difficult to define the characteristics which can be used as basis for defining these processes. At each period of time, different kinds of characteristics get appeared in human beings and on basis of these characteristics, some experts have classified stages of growth into four categories, namely :

(1) Infancy,

(2) Childhood,

(3) Adolescence, and

(4) Adulthood.

Human beings get transmitted to next stage in a natural way. However, these stages of growth does not consider to be water-tight, as sometimes it is found that features of one stage get transmitted in other stage also, the reason being that some fundamental traits take time to grow. Stages of development can be defined for human beings but it is not possible to do so for other living organisms. It is necessary to define different stages of development for human beings as they live in society and interact with other people.

Persons belonging to different stages possess different characteristics, which basically makes it clear that which person belongs to which category. To understand the concept of stages of growth and development, it is necessary to discuss all the stages as explained by experts, which are as follows :—

(1) Infancy

All living organisms possess the ability to produce or give birth to a new life. A new life take birth when a male and a female performs intercourse, because of which ovum gets united with spermatozoon. The seed that born in the womb of female gets sprout after a period of nine months. The period from conception to birth is called as pre-natal period of growth, and it is considered to be the most wonderful phenomena to study. During this period, fertilized egg gets turned into a child which is fully complete in anatomically sense. Child while remaining inside mother's womb perform various kinds of physiological functions, however, these all are indirect in nature. The most direct function, that is respiration, is performed when child gets out of his mother's womb. Various kinds of changes take place in child resting in mother's womb and various symptoms of growth begins to appear in child during this stage. The moment child comes out of mother's womb, he gets automatically included in category of infants. Child belonging to this stage have certain specific features, which can be discussed under following headings :—

i. Physical Features

All the organic parts of body which are required for biological activities are carried with body of child when he takes birth. Only those organs remain on the body which are present at time of birth, however, except teeth and sometime hair. All sense organs remain present on child's body and with time they all begin to function properly on their own. All brain cells remains in body of child and new born baby has a full grown nervous-system.

After birth, cells present in baby's body increase in size and number of axons also get increased because of which their brain also grow. After some time, their nervous-system become quite complex in nature. Body weight of baby after birth varies from 7½ pounds to 8 pounds, while height of his body is measured around 19½ inches. It is found that weight of baby boys is more than baby girls. Muscles of new born baby is soft and small. Muscles of hands, neck and arms seem to be less develop at time of birth. There seems lack of proportion among different parts of body. Eyes of new born baby remains so small that it seems that they cannot open them properly. They do not have much control over eye-movements and body parts movement. At the time of birth, pulse rate of infants vary from 130 to 150 beats per minute while after a few days, it gets decreased upto 118 beats per minute. A reduction take place in respiration rate which was around 40 at the time of birth, but decreases to 18 within few days.

Nervous system of infants has immature condition, because of which they find it difficult to move different organs of body in co-ordinated manner. When a stimulus is applied to any area of their body, there seems to be diffusion of energy in them. In such kind of situation, they move their entire body and not only that part where stimulus was applied.

It is wrong to expect that organs of infants will perform some special kind of functions on their own. It is after a long period of time that child begins to move different limbs of his body at his own will. At this age, children do not find to perform differentiated movements. Children of this age are capable of performing only reflexive activities. Even these activities can be performed only with limited organs of the body. All the activities are performed with unco-ordinated organs. In this state of age, children are considered no better than animals, as they do not have any mental qualities and as they cannot perform different activities on their own.

In a child's life, first two years play very crucial role, as possibilities of getting affected by special diseases remains high during this time. After a period of two years, he become able to perform various kinds of activities which he could not perform earlier. Physical growth takes place in similar manner in case of boys and girls. Various studies have proved that increase in weight take place more rapidly than height. However, with passage of time, these attributes begin to grow with different or at same pace. In the first year, bones elongation takes place rapidly, while in second year, rate of growth lowers down. Process of muscle development take place rapidly in first two years because of which child becomes able to perform various kinds of movements on his own. Now muscular system of baby develops as a result of which he begins to control almost all the organs of his body properly. Co-ordinated pattern of movement gets cleared as nervous system gets developed during this period. Till now, child begins to roll and crawl on his own. After sometime, he begins to walk on his own. After a long series of preparatory co-ordination, ability to maintain an upright posture gets developed in child. Movement patterns may vary from child to child, but it is certain that almost all the children can hold pencil or some like object properly after completion of one year.

Till the baby enters age of two, he begins to open various kinds of boxes and indulge himself in arranging boxes in specific manner. He perform various kinds of physical activities, but still they possess a rudimentary form. Child of this age group likes to indulge in all kinds of physical activities, as he obtains pleasure from these. After some time, all activities, which were rudimentary in the beginning, begin to possess definite form and seems more organised than before.

At the age of three, child indulge himself in various kinds of quick movements, e.g., running, jumping and bouncing. His pronunciation improves and he begins to pronounce even difficult words. He does not feel afraid of falling and even take part in risky activities.

Till now, muscles and bones present in his body get properly developed and he begins to hold heavy objects. For writing purpose, he makes use of his entire fore-arm as finer muscles of the fingers are not under his nervous control till now.

After crossing age of three, pace of growth lowers down and during this period, greater proportions get reflected in terms of height and weight. Some begins to recognise the child as mini adult. Now his bones have more hardness because of which his ability to lift heavy objects get developed and now they obtain a specific shape. He now indulge in various vigorous physical activities like skipping and galloping etc. Whenever he is provided with some rhythm, he begins to kick his leg or fling is arms. Now possibilities of getting affected by various diseases get reduced to a considerable extent.

ii. Mental Features

When a child is born, he possess of complete sense organs, but functionally, they are raw in nature. This can be proved by the fact that at time of birth, children do not recognise different kinds of colours. Skin of such children is so soft that it seems to be like cotton. New born baby is not developed psychologically as he does not have any individual experiences. Whatever a child experience in his environment, emotions of pleasure and pain get aroused during this age. Child begins to cry when his any need does not fulfilled properly. Emotion resulting from any kind of stimulus will be intensive and it will be very sudden.

Although new born babies possess the quality of responding emotionally, but they are not able to do so during this time as this quality exist in a non-developed state. No child can achieve emotional maturation without gratification of different kinds. During this age, people around child led the foundation on which structure of his personality rests. In the first two years, child begins to understand various things. By child completes 1 year of age, he begins to utter certain simple words, however, form of which does not seem to be very pure. On mental abilities of child depend the efficiency with which he builds his vocabulary store. In this respect, girls stand ahead of boys. In this aspect, various kinds of differences can be found among children.

With development of child, his emotional responses acquire a less diffuse state and they become more specialised in nature. Various specialised kind of emotions begin to develop in child. A child seems to be conversant with his environment till he reaches pre-school age. He begins to understand meaning of some abstract concepts and learns to express various kinds of feelings. He begins to count numbers and learn different incidence taking place some days before.

When children reach age of five, they become more emotional. Various kinds of fears enter into their mind and now they begin to laugh and cry on very small incidents. They try to imitate elders and does not like to remain in boundations in any way. They begin to over-estimate their energies and try to do things, which usually they cannot perform. A lot of aggression get developed in themselves, which get reflected very clearly in their acts. After attaining age of four, aggression found in children gets lower to some extent and in later parts of infancy, instinct of self-assertion becomes quite powerful. If seen mentally, child becomes self-possessive during this period and feels uncomfortable from interferences of others in his life.

Till this age, ability to concentrate on specific things and functions does not get developed in children and their interest keep on shifting from one activity to another. A lot of curiosity is found in him to know unknown things. Harsh punishments provided to children of this age group affects their mental make-up to a lot of extent and can direct their energies in negative direction. Child of this age group likes to spent time in company of other children, especially belonging to his age group. These children have their own liking and dislikings, on basis of which they choose different objects and activities for themselves.

(iii) Physical Activities

Children in this age group likes to participate in all kinds of physical activities. They do not require any kind of special objects to play with. They can use any valuable thing as their playing object. They like to throw all the things that come in front of them. Some children consider their toys as living and they begins to talk to them or behave with them as if they are living.

During this period, various external factors define the kind of physical activity in which children like to participate. It is very important to indulge children of this age group in appropriate physical activities as it is only during this time that fundamental human motor skills get established and developed in children. Some children like to participate in creative activities, while some of them like to take part in vigorous activities. Usually it is found that boys participate in active activities while girls like to take part in passive activities. Some of children like to make various kinds of objects from different things, like sand, mud and paper etc., thus indulge themselves in creative plays.

After some period, they like to participate in group activities where they can strive to perform well. The quality to obey someone's instructions get developed during this age in the children. They do not participate in complex kind of activities. They like to play only those games, in which they can perform their activities with freedom. They do not participate in game for long period of time, rather cut for intervals from short period of time. Generally the activities in which children of this age group participate are not organised by any rules and regulations. Every player creates his or her own rules and just try to imitate other players or some elder whom they seen performing the task.

(2) Childhood

A child is considered to be in his childhood, when he completes fourth year of life. This stage lasts until child does not complete age of twelve. During this period, process of growth take place with a uniform pattern. Some experts have divided this stage again into two sub-parts, namely, early childhood and later childhood. Early childhood has been explained by some experts as period of advancement, while period of later childhood has been explained as period of consolidation.

Till child attains age of three, process of growth take place with fast pace but then gradually this pace gets lowered down. Rate of growth again gets initiated when child attains age of six. After this, the rate lowers down and a kind of stability comes in this process. Later childhood is marked distinctively by this state of stability.

According to some experts, age of childhood can best be described as pseudo maturity prior to onset of puberty. By the age of twelve, all qualities get developed in child which help him to make adjustment in accordance with changed conditions. After sometime, process of growth seems to be stagnant and then period of consolidation sets into being. This period is consider very important for all the children as it is during this age that pre-natal experiences are being collected by them.

Today, through the evolution of preparatory schools, parents get their children admitted in the schools at onset of this period. Now, for the first time, he crosses jurisdiction of house and meets various children belonging to his age, which brings a magical transformation in his behaviour. Here for the first time, a kind of conflict is felt by him between forces of freedom and that of restraint. His behaviour gets modified to a lot of extent by social consciousness. Various kinds of social pressures lead to repression of various inner urges. At this age, process of formal education begins because of which it is considered to be very important stage for children. It is said that all the behaviours which a child learns or acquired in this age dominate him throughout the life. Parents and teachers begin to meticulous about daily habits of child and if he performs any act wrongly, then he is provided with appropriate punishment.

Physical Features : Various kinds of physical changes take place in physical attributes of children belonging to this age group. Around two to three inches increase take place in their height while their body weight increases from three to five Ibs. Physically, boys seem to be in more stronger position in comparison to girls. Height and weight, both qualities develop during this period, however, proportion of this process varies from child to child.

An important change taking place in child of this age group is that permanent teeth gets grown in place of milk teeth, because of which his facial structure gets changed to a lot of extent. By such kind of change, some children feel confident while shame is being felt by some. They lips get fill out and size of nose becomes large. Different limbs of body acquire shape during this period and they acquire a totally new outlook. Almost all parts of body acquire broadness and become wider than earlier. Greater increase in size of legs and arms take place during this period. In late childhood period, pace of growth taking place in feet and hands remain very low, but it has been found that size of girl's hands and legs remains less than boy's. During this period, children seem to be growing without any proportion.

Mental Features : At this age, a child gets mentally developed to a considerable extent. He now becomes able to think about some facts independently and learns to visualise various aspects of anything even in absence of that object in physical form. Liking to indulge in activities with children of same age group increases and by this, they learn various new medium of expressions. He begins to read various kinds of books, because of which his vocabulary store gets rich to a lot of extent.

Till now, all the children establishes relationship with other people living in society, and especially with children belonging to their own age group. They try to understand social norms and become very curious to find out the reasons of someone's odd behaviour. Feelings of likeness and dislikeness gets aroused in children of this age group and they feel more attracted towards those persons whom they like. Children in this age group have a very fantastic attitude and they live in an imaginary life, which is quiet different from real world. They begin to understand various kinds of problems arising in different areas of life and also get worried by these problems. In the beginning, they try to solve all kinds of problems without help of others, but at last when realise that it is not possible for them, seek help of parents or friends. During this period, an emotion which dominate children is anger. Sometimes, their level of anger reaches more than expected. Another emotion which develops in children of this age group is jealousy, which may arise against children of their own age group. They begin to tease those children against whom they feel jealousy. They expressions become more intense and sober than before and they like to spent most of their time with children of their own age.

Development of Motor Skills : It is found from various studies that children belonging to this age group are full of energy and vigour. They like to participate in energetic and especially in outdoor activities. The level of success which a child will attain during this period gets determined to a lot of extent by the manner in which he acquires proper motor skills. Various kinds of motor skills are acquired by children specially during this period. They begin to move different parts of body while maintain co-ordination and balance.

Due of various factors, level of motor skill development can remain lower in children of this age group, because of which their performance level will also remain lower. Depending upon the performance level a child attains, various kinds of attitude gets developed in the children of this age. Feeling of inferiority and superiority develops in them during this age. Their liking to participate in group or social activities gets lowered down and now they feel shy while taking part in such activities. However, such kind of feeling do not get developed in all the children, but in which it gets, they cannot turn out to be outstanding players in any activity.

Whether children become proficient in motor skills or not depends to a lot of extent on various factors, some of which are kind of surroundings or environment provided, kind of people surrounding them and attitude of parents towards them. Some parents do mistake of pressurising the children to participate in activities in which they do not have any interest. Such kind of pressure may generate harmful effects. To attain accuracy in performance, it becomes necessary for the players to do continuous practice. Thus, children of this age group like to indulge themselves in more organised and proper activities.

By the time children attains age of six, they become crazy for participating in vigorous activities. He remains filled with thirst for action. Now he becomes able to make use of different parts of his body while maintaining equilibrium among them. He love to participate in dangerous activities, because of which he often gets rebuke from parents and teachers. Child does not like to keep his body in rest position. He wants to indulge himself continuously in risky ventures and now likes to participate in complex activities.

Physical Activities : Likeness for taking part in physical activities take different shapes in different children belonging to this age group. Generally it is seen that likeness to participate in physical activities gets reduced or lowered among children of this age group, however who possess it, show great vigour and vitality in play activities. Today, studies have become so stressful that children do not find time to participate in physical activities. Time of school-child gets restricted to some specific activities, because of which tendency to participate in physical activities get lowered.

Children of this age group likes to participate in vigorous kinds of activities. Keeping in view the abilities of children, various kinds of physical activities are being organised in school but students who do not get such kind of opportunities have to indulge themselves in non-organised activities. Those activities should be organised to more extent, in which gross body movements are being used by players. Such kind of activities should be organise for children upto ten year of age. For children of this age group, those activities should be organised to a minimum level which involve endurance. Teacher should attempt to develop qualities of endurance and speed in the children.

c. Adolescence : This is a Latin word, which means grow to maturity. Initial stage of adolescence is considered to be puberty. Period of puberty can be considered a period in which a child gets entered into the phase of adolescence. During this period, a child gets converted into adult in a natural way, because of which this period is considered to be very important in life of a human being.

Stage of adolescence begins to puberty, but last until child does not get developed fully. It commences with end of late childhood. A person is considered to be in his adolescent when he completes the age of twelve. Various kinds of changes can take place in children belonging to this age group. The age in which a person gets into adolescent period varies from person to person, which normally depends on various factors. Girls enter into this period before boys. Various geographical, nutritional and socio-economic factors determine the time span of this period.

This stage of a human being is considered as most critical one as it is in this period that it gets determined that what kind of personality a person will have and what attitude he will have towards various things. During this period, life seems to be uncontrollable to the person and he finds it difficult to keep his life under control and equilibrium. Every aspects of growth begins to vary during this period. Various kinds of changes take place in physique and mental set-up of persons belonging to this age group, some of the important features which define the person in this stage can be explained in following manner :—

i. Physical Features: When a child gets entered in stage of puberty, tremendous acceleration take place in physical growth. There seems a considerable change in physical proportion of his body. Primary and secondary sex characteristics begins to develop more prominently. All the features which define sex of people seems clearly apparent. Now children are not recognised as children, but as mature beings. They are not expected to behave in childish way.

All the body parts of children gets developed to fuller extent and they seems to attain proper shape. Various factors affect sexual maturity taking place in children of this age group. Process of maturation take place early in girls than in comparison to boys. Various kinds of changes take place in facial make-over of children, which work as evidences of matureness.

Boys get beared on their faces while cycle of menstruation gets begin in girls during this age. After attainment of these processes, process of physical growth either lowers down or stops entirely. Now girls become capable of reproduction and they get attracted towards persons of opposite sex. During childhood, sex-impulse lie dormant in children, but as they enter into this stage, this impulse gets violent, because of which it becomes very difficult for persons to control themselves. By the time children enter into this age group, they become wholly developed physically and now level of energy also gets increased. Now they can indulge themselves in vigorous activities and even can perform for long period of times. Thus, various kinds of physical changes take place in children during this period and their personality get set-up in this period.

ii. Mental Features: Children belonging to this age group have a mature mental zone and till now their intelligence horizon gets broaden to a lot of extent. Now they can understand all the concepts relating to their life or life of others. They can even understand new concepts, about which they do not have any prior knowledge or information.

Generally children belonging to this age group develops their likeness and dislikeness and on this basis chose to participate in different kinds of activities. Some of them like to participate in physical activities, while some like to get new information through different sources. Now they do not live in self-created world but understands harsh realities of world. Mentally, children belonging to this age group have matured because of which they can take various decisions of their life independently. They possess the quality to assess all things from various perspective and like to take part in those activities in which they are required to make use of their mental capacities.

If seen from emotional point of view, adolescents have maturer ground and now they know how to control different kinds of emotions. They react to different situations in appropriate kind, but sometimes they feel themselves caught in emotional turmoil because of which they commit some mistakes in life but they begin to learn something from their mistakes. Now they do not seem to be feared from risky activities while they like to do so. In some adolescents, curiosity to explore various unexplored fields and concepts get increased while their attitude towards sex gets changed and they try to indulge themselves in more sources from where they can get information relating to healthful sex.

iii. Physical Activities : As adolescents attain physical and mental matureness because of which they attain the ability to perform various kinds of difficult and complex skills easily. Sports coach should understand the fact that they are full of energy because of which they should be indulged in those activities where they can utilise their energy properly.

Important Points to be Kept in Mind

While creating programme, it is very necessary for the coach to keep in mind the age group to which players belong as all the children belonging to different age groups have varying physical and mental capacities. Not only this, their liking and disliking also differ. If programme is being made for girl children then they should be provided with different place as some of them may feel shy to practice skills in front of others. However, with development, their level of shyness gets decreased.

Coach should understand that all children like to participate in physical activities because of which he should provide more time for practice purpose. He should not give more importance to theory of game as it can result in boredom in children. In childhood, players should be provided utmost care and sympathy however, level of care can be reduced for adolescents.

Students in childhood stage can be indulged in non-organised sports activities, however, adolescents should be indulged in proper or well-organised sports and they should be provided with standard equipments, so that they can turn out be fruitful players for the organisation and can take part in national and international games.

INFLUENCE OF HEREDITY AND ENVIRONMENTAL FACTORS ON PROCESSES OF GROWTH AND DEVELOPMENT

Various biological and psychological factors affect the heredity and environment of an individual. Different opinions are being provided by different experts. Experts who believe in biological scientists advocate in favour of various inherited qualities for an integral development of a student. According to such experts, personality of an individual do not change and they remain as they are however, behaviour of students or any individual can get change because of the various persons they come into contact with. When the question of all around development of an individual arises, importance of certain innate qualities cannot be ignored. Qualities of aggression, self-preservation are such kinds of innate qualities. Such qualities are inherited biologically and they affect an individual's personality to a lot of extent.

If viewed according to this aspect, it will realise that utmost importance is being provided to inherited traits and environmental factors have been ignored to a lot of extent. There are some experts who criticise this concept on this basis. Such experts do not accept the superiority of inherited traits in comparison to environmental factors. Such experts are firm believers of the notion that it is not possible to create any player, but players are born with such qualities which help them in becoming outstanding players. Quality and performance of players can be only improved with the help of various services, like diet controls and proper motivation.

After analysing both the arguments, it will be realised that an extreme approach in favour of heredity and environment has been adopted by both kinds of experts. On the basis of both kinds of arguments, it can be said that heredity and environment plays an important role in shaping the personality of an individual, thus man is actually a produce of heredity and environment. Sports is a social institution and biological necessity, because of which a sportsman should be considered as an blend or mixture of the two. A sportsman get not affected only by biological factors but sociological forces also play an important role in affecting him. In addition to these, various other factors play a very important role in shaping the personality of an individual. Such factors include social practices, religious attitudes and type of school in which student gets education.

Today, the function of physical educator is not only concerned with imparting education relating to various activities to the students, but they also provide guidance to them in different kinds of personal matters.

Thus it can be said that it is not possible to bring any

kind of change in the genetic make up of any individual, but it is possible to develop these inherited potentials to a lot of extent. This thing can be done by providing him a cordial environment in which he can easily and without any problem bring a kind of development in his inherited factors. It is in the very effective manner that factors of heredity and environment influence processes of growth and development.

Age and Sex Differences in Concern with Physical Activities and Sports

Today, in our country, we find that at various levels of education boys and girls get education simultaneously, and it is not possible to appoint separate physical educators for both kinds of students. Physical educators should kept in mind that boys and girls are different from each other in various respects. Various kinds of important differences are being found in the students of both the sexes.

Various kinds of differences take place after the stage of puberty. Upto the puberty stage, hardly any difference is seen between boys and girls but as they cross this stage, one can very clearly view the differences that emerge in them. While formulating physical education programme for the students of both sexes, physical educator should kept in his mind all these marked differences. These differences not only result because of various biological factors, but various social factors also play an important role in bringing such kind of differences. For this reason, physical educators should construct separate programmes for boys and girls, otherwise, it will not bring any kind of beneficial results.

Some kind of Differences in Males and Females

Some of the mark differences which are being found

between a girl and boy are as follows :—

a. Rate of growth of the students of both the sexes is not same. They do not grow at the same pace. In the age of early adolescence, girls grow faster in comparison to boys but their rate of growth diminishes after the age of 14. In case of boys, they grow with a slow pace before the adolescence age, but their this rate diminishes after the age of 14 to 16 years.

b. After crossing the age of 14, girls students find it difficult to run faster without any problem the reason of which is that they have broader and shallow pelvis. In case of boys, this kind of problem does not arise because they have narrow pelvis in relation to girls and does not find it difficult to run at any rate.

c. Generally it is found that height of girls remain smaller or shorter in comparison to boys. They can attain height only in early age of maturity, but boys can attain height even in later stages of maturity.

d. Girls also find it difficult to jump properly because they have large body and shorter limbs, which makes their centre of gravity low. In comparison to girls, boys have shorter trunk and long legs. They have a high centre of gravity which provide them with an unstable position. Because of this reason, boys do not find any problem in jumping events.

e. Girls have smaller heart but a faster pulse rate. This is the main reason why the pulse rate of the girl players increases in the beginning of exercise, but slower down after the exercise. Because of more muscle tissues, boys have larger heart in comparison to girls and have better blood circulation because of which in the beginning of exercise, they do not get tired easily.

f. Girls cannot perform better than boys in the field of pulling and punching activities because they have less muscular strength. In comparison to them, boys have more muscular power and because of which they can perform activities of punching, kicking and putting better or efficiently.

g. Reaction and movement time of girls is very slow in comparison to boys.

h. One of an important change that can take place only in girls is the beginning of menstruation cycle. This cycle results because of biological activities. In boys, this kind of no such biological activity take place.

i. Girls use upper part of their chest to breath more shallowly while boys breaths deeply in comparison to girls.

All the differences mentioned above affect performances of girls and boys students to a lot of extent. Physical educator should have a thorough knowledge of all these differences. From the above discussion, one can easily predict that girls are being placed at an inferior position in comparison to boys because of various biological factors. Age and sex differences are the very important aspects, which a physical educator should kept in mind while preparing programmes for students of both the sexes.

Different Phases of Age

The process of growth do not take place with the same pace in different age groups. We find varying degree of changes or fluctuations in the rate of this process. In a school, a large number of students get education and they all differ in various respect from each other. A physical educator has to provide education or training to all the students with varying differences. Because of the differences in physical and mental abilities of students, it become a difficult task for the physical educator to provide education to all of them in the same manner and at the same place.

It is indicated by the processes of growth and development that a child gets developed through various stages and one can find various kinds of differences in all the stages. Various kinds of changes are being found in an infant and an adolescent. Various criterion can be used to classify the students into various groups. For classifying the students, it is not necessary to have proper knowledge of their age in terms of month and years. One can easily find required data from register of the school. In our country, some people do not get registration of the birth of their child because of which, sometimes the problem of identifying their age arises. In such kind of situations, the criteria that is used to classify the students is their developmental characteristics. All these kinds of developmental characteristics provide different kinds of age, which play an important role in determining the personality of a student.

Different kinds of age, which result from various developmental characteristics are as follows :—

a. Anatomical Age,

b. Chronological Age,

c. Mental Age, and

d. Physiological Age

Anatomical Age

The process which brings a kind of development in the skeletal system of an individual is known as anatomical age. In determining the anatomical age of a person, quality of bone structure plays an important role. To determine the extent or rate of development taking place in skeletal system, technique of X-ray is being used.

Skeletal development of a child is affected to a lot of extent by the kind of food he or she takes. Thus, the level of nutrition in the foods of child plays an important role in determining the rate of development of skeletal in an individual.

What kind of weight exercises should be practised by the different students, this important thing is determined by considering the anatomical age of the child. Some children have strong skeleton while some have soft. Children with soft skeleton should not be allowed to practice heavy exercises, as it can create various kinds of problems in their skeleton systems.

Chronological Age

Age of a person that is determined by the day on which he was born and the time of this occurrence. Thus that age of a person which can be recorded in terms of years, months and days is termed as chronological age. To calculate this kind of age, the day on which child takes birth and the day on which he dies are being taken into consideration.

Generally, this kind of age is being used to classifying a students in various categories. To decide whether a student should be included in the junior, sub-junior or senior teams, this kind of age is considered.

The manner in which development in one student take place differ from other students. Various kinds of changes are being viewed in various individuals in terms of physical qualities because individual rate of growth of each individual differ from each other. It is because of difference in the rate of growth with leads a kind of difference in mental ability of different students. Generally, for classifying students into various categories, their chronological age is being taken into account.

Mental Age

To the mental development of a child, his mental age is concerned. Mental development can be considered a process of mental maturation taking place in an individual. One thing should be kept in mind that there lies a lot of difference between physical and mental maturity. There is generally no relationship between mental maturity and physical development. We can find various individuals who have grown up in terms of physique, but not have attained a developed state of brain.

Various kinds of psychological tests are being used to detect the mental age of students. If any student is physically developed, he should not be considered mentally mature. Some children becomes maturer in terms of their mental abilities earlier and some later. Mental age of students can be determined with the help of various psychological tests. By knowing the level of mental development of a student, a teacher can very easily and properly construct the kind of physical education programme that suits him. Age groups should be formed, the basis of which should be body structure of students, their standards and objectives. Principle of homogeneity should be followed in order to classify the students into different categories. Same technique or programme should not be designed for all the students because every student differ from each other in various respect. Children of different age group should be trained differently and competitions between students of different age groups should not be organised. If matching is done properly, it provides a kind of confidence to the students and chances of their becoming injured decreases to a lot of extent.

Physiological Age

Physiological capabilities of students affect their age to a lot of extent. Generally, it is concerned with puberty. While calculating the age of a child, secretion of hormones from various glands and functional conditions of the organs should be taken into account. In case of girls, this age can be calculated on the basis of set of menstruation cycles, while in case of boys, growth of hair in the armpit can be taken or considered the base.

If age of the students is known to the physical educator, it becomes easy for him to prepare work schedules for different students. Some students with advanced chronological age are found to be immature in terms of physiological terms. This is an important factor which obstructs the physical activity programme to a lot of extent. Physiological age of children should be taken into account while working out the activity loads for them. Only those activities should be practised or used which suit the physiological age of the students. Children, having similar physiological age should be provided training at the same time. Only those children should be allowed to play with each other who belong to same physiological age group.

Thus, there are various kinds of ages through which various children passes from. The age in years, months and days of a child may not compare with the age of his development. Anatomical or physiological items in the individual may run ahead or lag behind in development for the normal age. The ossification of bones indicates anatomical age. This may be determined by the x-ray. Physiological age represents a functional condition and in relation to chronological age, may present marked variation.

Chronological age is a poor measure of capacity in either boys or girls. Physiological maturity represented in sexual development may range over a period of four to five years. Maturity may come at 10½ years or not until 16½ years. The median age for this development is between 13½ and 14 years. Early maturity is not a sign of poor health. Tall girls mature generally earlier than short ones.

Physical education should take into account physiological age in conduct of activities. Physiological age has significance for physical education. Children tend to play with others of their same physiological age and they select activities suited to their stage of development. Girls are older physiologically than boys. Moreover, early or late maturity of youths may present adjustment problems of which the teacher should be aware. Large size in a girl often complicates the posture problem, and if the breasts are well developed, this sign of maturity may lead to a postural stoop and a marked decrease of interest in sports activities. Small size in a boy is likewise contrary to the ideals of the culture and may produce emotional problems of compensatory character.

Different Kinds of Bodies

Different biological, psychological, sociological, and cultural factors effect physical characteristics to a lot of extent and this fact result differences in varying degree in the body type of different individuals. From ancient times, it is believed that an individual's body type is related to various factors, such as his health, immunity for diseases and physical performance. Taking this thinking as a base, various experts have various body structures in different categories.

For all the individuals, it is very important to study the kind of physique. This concept is related to understanding of various concepts, like physical and mental state of the individual and his emotional condition. A physical educator have to provide education to different kinds of students, for this reason, he should have thorough knowledge relating to the physique pattern of all the students. With the help of such knowledge, he will be able to do his function of imparting knowledge to students very easily. Not only this, with the help of such knowledge, he can, without any problem, maintain discipline in the class and can classify the students into different categories.

Information relating to physique of undergraduate students of physical education should be get from their parents. It is believed by some experts that human beings differ from each other to such an extent that it is not possible to categorise them into two or three categories. According to these experts, human bodies are made up of some primary components, and to classify the body types into different categories, these components should be used as the base. Endomorph, Ectomorph and Mesomorph are these primary components which make up a human body.

Endomorph

This is one kind of body structure. People with such

structure of body are able to digest the hard food, through which they get the energy. They have round heads, broad face and square jaw. Their abdomen is large in size. Size of their neck is generally short. They have fatty breasts. They have broad feet with low arch. Their skin is of hairy and thick type. Their buttocks are heavy in weight. They broad palms and their fingers are short in length.

Such kind of people over-estimate their abilities. They generally remains in relaxed and good mood. They get bore very easily from routine work. In various kinds of sports activities, such people take part.

Ectomorph

People with such body build have poor digestive system and have less energy output. Their body structure seems to be very delicate. They have small face and a sharp nose. Neck of such kind of people is quite slender and they have long arms. Buttocks and legs of such kind of people is quite thin. They have long feet. Their skin is soft and have a lots of hair. Their vital capacity is quite low, but they are tall. They do functions or various works with low speed.

Under-estimation of their abilities is an important feature of such kind of people. They are ambition, but lack self-confidence. They try to solve various kinds of problems at their mental level and make use of their energy to a limited extent. They feel irritated and tensed in very simple problems or conditions. The kind of sports activities in which they like to part includes : Basketball, Volleyball and Running.

Mesomorph

Such kind of people have medium height. They are generally considered athletic type persons. Their bones are large in size and prominent in nature. They have long face bones and their calvin bones are quite heavy. They have large abdomen and low waist. Their buttocks are heavy in weight and they have heavy fore legs. They have rough skin. In nature, they like to dominate others, are full of energy and like to task various kinds of risks in their life. They can make decisions very quickly and can handle difficult problems on their own. They have a direct forward nature and have a clear mind.

Thus, various kinds of body types are being classified into above mentioned categories, but it is not necessary that only these categories can provide authentic information about the bodily structure of an individual. For this reason, while taking any kind of decision, it is very necessary to take into account various kinds of other factors, like strength, skill, physical fitness and interest of the student.

5

PSYCHOLOGICAL FOUNDATION OF PHYSICAL EDUCATION

INTRODUCTION

Man is considered the most complicated and superior creature of God. It is the complicated process which God has used in creating man which has given the nature of complications to all kinds of activities which human beings perform. It has remained an important subject of research that why do the human beings and animals behave in the manner they behave.

The credit to originate the concept of philosophy goes to some Greek Philosophers. Term psychology is composed of two distinct words, namely, the psyche and logos. Psyche implies the soul while logic to study something. Thus, when both these two words, with distinct meanings join each other, a new meaning derives from this joining procedure and this new meaning is the "Study of Souls or Mind of human beings".

According to various Greek philosophers, human beings perform various kinds of mental activities with the help or by using their soul. They held that principle of life is the soul of human beings or all the living creatures. Because it is not possible to study one's soul, because of which experts have defined psychology as that branch of study which deals with mind of an individual.

For the first time, use of this word was done by Rudolf Goeckel in the year 1590. He used it in context of study of an individual's mind. It is not an easy task to study someone's mind. Even it is not as simple to define the concept of mind. Various research works have been conducted which are concerned with the actions and thinking of human beings. Some philosophers consider human soul and mind two different structures, which affect each other to a lot of extent.

It was declared by two German scientists that it is possible to study physical processes which underlay mental activities in the mid 1800's. World first psychology laboratory was founded by Wilhelm Wundt in the year 1875. Credit to publish the first journal of psychology also goes to Wilhelm Wundt.

Later, psychology was defined as description and explanation of state of consciousness of an individual by William James. To establish psychology as a distinct field, works of William James and Wundt helped to a lot of extent. To do this work, both the psychologists used the different methods. To understand the conscious mind, Wundt broke down the mental processes into various parts and employed the method of introspection to analyse the fact that how these factors are inter-related with each other. In this method, sub-conscious and un-conscious activities of the mind were not taken into account, on the ground of which, this method was being rejected and did not get much popularity and success. Introspection method was also considered to an unscientific and subjective method for which psychologists do not favour to employ it. To solve this problem, John Watson and his followers did a lot of work.

Watson and his followers concentrated on the behavioural aspect of an individual and they provide the new definition of psychology as study of behaviour. According to William McDoughall, Psychology is a science whose objective is to give us proper understanding of control of behaviour of an individual as a whole. He also believed that in shaping up an individual's behaviour, environment plays an important role. This kind of thinking became popular with the works of Russian psychologist Ivan P. Pavlov. Later it was realised by some experts that conditioning can play an important role in influencing the human behaviour.

According to Gestalt movement, behaviour of an individual should be studied as an organised pattern and not as a separate incidents of stimulus and response. Definition provided by Watson is considered incomplete as it did not include or take into account the mental process of the individual.

It was in the year 1900 that a new dimension was being added to the field of psychology by Sigmund Freud through his psycho-analysis approach. It was stated by him that it is not possible to understand an individual's overt behaviour without taking into account his unconscious springs of motivation. Behaviour is determined by powerful inner forces was the basis of psycho-analysis theory. These forces are situated or have their place in unconscious mind.

From time to time, various experts have devoted their time on working on various aspects of psychology, and as a result of all these studies or researches, concept of psychology is keep on changing its face. Today, or the according to the modern concept of psychology, it takes into account everything or factor that contribute in any way to the understanding of an individual behaviour. Thus, all the factors, which help in understanding the behaviour of an individual are constitutes of psychology. This is the modern concept of psychology, which is based not on imagination but on reality. In this approach, greater emphasis is being placed on concrete aspect of behaviour of the individual. This kind of approach give rise to the concepts of humanistic psychology. There are various important human psychologists, like Abraham H. Maslow and Carl R. Rogers, who have contributed a lot in the field of psychology. These psychologists believed that in controlling individuals, their values play an important role. To make various kinds of choices, environment plays an important role, but function of other factors is also very important in this respect.

The main objective of humanistic psychology is to help human beings to function in such a manner and they can get good results and can also fulfil their needs. Concept of trans-personal Psychology came into existence after the concept of Humanistic Psychology. Trans-personal psychology deals with the area that how human beings feel in different states of awareness. One of a recently developed concept in the psychology is Cognitive psychology, which takes into account higher cognitive abilities and capacities of human beings which help them to adapt themselves according to the changed environment.

Concept of psychology in modern times considers the principles mentioned above as basis to a lot of extent. According to some psychologists, modern psychology is the investigation of behaviour of human beings and other living creatures and it is also related to the mental and physiological processes which are being associated with their behaviour Inspite of development of various kinds of techniques, there is not much marked difference in the meaning and definition of psychology. Thus, the concept of psychology is same today as it was in earlier days. Even today, it is considered that branch of science which deals with behaviour of human beings and other living creatures.

PSYCHO-PHYSICAL ACTIVITY AND PHYSICAL EDUCATION

There are confusion prevalent for years between many educationists, physical education teachers and psychologists in collaborating and relating physical education as mind-body or muscle-mind. The scientists however solved these disputes explaining that mind without physical body and body without a mind can not exist.

Generally, an individual thinks with his mind and exercises control over his body. Different parts of body carry out their functions with directions from mind. Nature has co-ordinated the mutual actions of mind and body in a very orderly manner. By this way we may say that our behaviour has two directions: -

1. Internal or mental
2. External or physical

1. Internal or mental: Analysis of the situations by mental faculties.

2. External or physical : To perform the work efficiently by physical organs.

It is observed that mental state of any individual effect his physical state while his physical situation too fully effects his mental state both are vice-versa and inter-related.

Everything that happens in your life, and everything that happens in your body, begins with something happening in your consciousness. Your consciousness is who you are, your experience of Being.

You decide what ideas to accept and which to reject. You decide what to think, and you decide what to feel. When these decisions leave you with residual stress, you experience the stress as if in your physical body.

We know that stress creates symptoms. The interesting question is, "Which stress creates which symptoms?" When we are able to quantify this process, we are then able to see the body as a map of the person's consciousness, and relate particular symptoms to particular stresses and particular ways of being, in the same way that Type "A" Behavior has been able to be associated with heart disease.

To understand this map, we must first orient ourselves to the idea that the causes of symptoms are within. While it's true that germs cause disease and accidents cause injuries, it is also true that this happens in accord with what is happening in the consciousness of the person involved.

Germs are everywhere. Why are some people affected and not others? Something different is happening in their consciousness. Why do some patients in hospitals respond better to treatment than others? They have different attitudes. Something different is happening in their consciousness When someone is injured in an "accident," why is it that a very specific part of the body is affected, and that it is the same part that has had habitual problems? Is that an "accident," or is there a pattern and an order to the way things happen in our bodies?

Your consciousness, your experience of Being, who you really are, is energy. We can call it "Life Energy" for now. This energy does not just live in your brain; it fills your entire body. Your consciousness is connected to every cell in your body. Through your consciousness, you can communicate with every organ and every tissue, and a number of therapies are based on this communication with the organs which have been affected by some kind of symptom or disorder.

This energy which is your consciousness, and which reflects your state of consciousness, can be measured through the process known as Kirlian photography. When you take a Kirlian photograph of your hand, it shows a certain pattern of energy. If you take a second photograph while imagining that you are sending love and energy to someone you know, there will be a different pattern of energy shown on the Kirlian photograph. Thus, we can see that a change in your consciousness creates a change in the energy field that is being photographed, which we call the aura.

This energy field shown in the Kirlian photographs has been quantified, so that when there are "holes" in particular parts of the energy field, these are said to correspond to particular weaknesses in specific parts of the physical body. The interesting thing about this is that the weakness shows up in the energy field before there is ever any evidence of it on the physical level.

Thus, we have an interesting direction of manifestation shown through what we have described.

A change of consciousness creates a change in the energy field.

A change in the energy field happens before a change in the physical. The direction of manifestation is from the consciousness, through the energy field, to the physical body.

When we look at things in this way, we see that it is not the physical body creating the energy field, the aura, but rather the aura or energy field that is creating the physical body. What we see as the physical body is the end result of a process that begins with the consciousness.

When someone makes a decision that leaves them with stress, creating a blockage in the energy field with a sufficient degree of intensity, this creates a symptom on the physical level. The symptom speaks a certain language, which reflects the idea that we each create our own reality. When the symptom is described from that point of view, the metaphoric significance of the symptom becomes clear. Thus, instead of saying, "I can't see," the person would have to say, "I have been keeping myself from seeing something." If they cannot walk, they would have to say, "I have been keeping myself from walking away from something." And so on.

We must understand that there are no accidents and no coincidences. Things do happen according to a pattern and order. We can say that we have an inner guidance system, a connection to our Higher Self, or our Inner Being, or whatever name we choose to give this Higher Intelligence. This inner guidance system functions through what we call our intuition, or our instinct. It speaks a very simple language. Either it feels good, or it doesn't. All the rest is just politics.

We are told we should move with what feels good, and do not do what doesn't feel good to us. We are told to trust this inner voice. When we don't follow this inner voice we feel tension. We feel not-good.

Then, the voice must get louder. The next level of communication is through the emotions. As we move more and more in the direction that feels not-good, we experience more and more emotions that feel not-good, and at some point we can say, "I should have listened to myself when I thought to move in the other direction." That meant that we heard the inner voice. Otherwise, we could not have said, "I should have listened." If we make the decision we know is the right one for us, and therefore change direction, there is a release of tension, we feel better, and we know we are again on the right track.

If we continue to move in the direction that feels not-good, the communication reaches the physical level. We create a symptom, and the symptom speaks a language which reflects the idea that we each create our own reality. When we describe the symptom from that point of view, we can understand the message. If we change our way of being, we have received the message, and the symptom has no further reason for being. It is able to be released, according to whatever we allow ourselves to believe is possible. If we created the symptom with a decision, we are also able to release it with a decision.

As an hypothesis, we can imagine that someone makes a decision that it is not a good idea to express what they want. From that moment, whenever there is something they want, they keep themselves from expressing it, and therefore from having what they want. That feels not-good. The tension grows. They feel more and more not-good as they keep themselves from expressing what they want and not having it.

Eventually, something happens to create a symptom on the physical level, and their right arm is affected. It could have happened through falling from a ladder, or in an automobile accident, or by pinching a nerve in the neck, or by "sleeping in a draft."

Something had to happen on the physical level to create the symptom, in order to give the person the message on the physical level about what they had been doing to themselves. We do to ourselves literally what we have been doing to ourselves figuratively.

The effect is that the person cannot move their arm. They are keeping themselves from reaching for something, and since it is the right arm, on the "will" side of the body, they are keeping themselves from reaching for or going for what they want. They have been giving themselves reasons to not believe that they could have what they want.

When they begin to do something different in their consciousness, they notice that something different begins to happen with their arm, and the symptom is able to be released.

UNDERSTANDING THE MEANING OF LEARNING

Human beings can adapt themselves in according to the conditions in which they are forced to live. It is not an easy task to survive or live in diverse conditions or environment. For this difficult task, human beings have developed various skills, which are intellectual and social in nature. Human beings develop these skills with the process of learning. It is a biological necessity for all the human beings to learn different skills or things from time to time.

Learning is a process with the help of which various kinds of changes or modifications take place in the behaviour of an individual. Process of learning results in acquiring new knowledge and skills. These changes or modifications have a nature of permanency. With the help of learning process, various kinds of changes in mental, social and physical domain can be found in human beings. Because of this reason, as a result of learning, not only motor skills of individuals get affected, but it also affects to a lot of extent their behavioural attitudes and social values.

In psychology, learning possess an important place. That process which helps in bringing various kinds of changes in behaviour of individuals is termed as learning. These kind of changes can result from various personal experiences and also by practice. All kinds of responses that an individual makes according to the environment are considered behaviour. Organisms of human body tries to react according to the environment and they adjust themselves accordingly. When the organs react to the environment, there arises a kind of reaction between organism and environment. This reaction is known as experience. The behaviour of an individual is affected to a lot of extent by the kind of environment he or she receives. If a child learns in normal behaviour, he will learn normal social behaviour while a child who learns in an unfavourable environment, will learn anti-social behaviour only.

It is not an easy task to give proper definition of the concept of learning as it is a very wide concept. All the activities and experiences which affect an individual in any way are included in it. Learning is not a process of short duration. It lasts for life time. Every day and every minute, human beings experiences different or new things and on the basis of their experiences, they try to modify their behaviour.

Learning in Physical Education

All kinds of changes that are concerned with the player's method of practising, participating and performing are considered to be occurred as a result of learning. When we talk about learning in physical education, it implies various kinds of changes that place in the behaviour of players or students taking part in any kind of physical activity. All those changes that take place in players as a result of observation, experience or practice are considered the result of learning. Accumulating new knowledge, improving the skill and solving some problem relating specifically to some aspect of the sport are main aspects of learning in physical education. Every individual learns in his life and it is by the quality of his learning that the mode of his behaviour gets affected. Learning is not only found in formal form, but it can take place in informal forms. All the phases of life get influenced by learning. Various kinds of good qualities get developed in human beings because of learning. Learning has various different implications, which make it a very complicated phenomenon.

Fundamental Rules of Learning

Although, learning can be in the formal and in informal manners, but some experts have stated that there are some rules or laws on the basis of which process of learning takes place. These rules are the working principles for the process of learning and they should be taken into account by the physical educators while imparting training or knowledge to the students. These rules specify the conditions or circumstances in which the process of learning should be carried out.

Some of the fundamental rules of learning are as follows :—

a. Rule of exercise,

b. Rule of readiness, and

c. Rule of effect.

Rule of Exercise

This rule is based on the notion that a man becomes perfect by practising on a continuance basis. The reaction becomes automatic, when an individual repeat something again and again. Principles of exercise and of practice or repetition are involved in this rule.

This rule is based on the belief that an individual can retain or remember only that thing which he repeats again and again. If he does not make use of anything, he will forget it after a limited period of time. Doing on continuance basis is very important for remembering something. No student or player can perform any skill properly if he does not practice it on continuance basis.

With the continuance practice, various kinds of changes take place in respect of development of skills, better coordination and less expenditure of energy. Distance between stimulus and response become more pronounced as a result of continuance practice. Unplanned or unco-ordinated practice do not bring any kind of fruitful results, but it is only with the help of well co-ordinated practice that proper results can be obtained. Such kind of practice helps in affecting various phases of learning processes. When the goals are set in advance, with the help of practice of skills on repetitions basis, student can achieve the goals quite easily and in minimum time.

Rule of Readiness

A human being learns something more quickly and effectively with the help of readiness. No one· can get desires goals if students are not willing to participate in the sports and they do it just because of some compulsion or pressure. If they are not willing to learn something, no one can teach them. In this respect, one of an important rules of learning is rule of readiness.

The word mindset mentions the preparatory attitude. If in reality learning process should be used, it is very necessary that the student or the individual should be physically, mentally and emotionally matured. Physical educators should encourage the students in such a way that they got attracted towards various sports activities.

Before actually participating in the sports, students should be provided sufficient time in which they can practice certain warm up exercises. Warm up exercises help in preparing the muscular system of the body to practice difficult or vigorous activities.

Rule of Effect

This rule is also known as rule of satisfaction. Learning process gets enhanced to a lot of extent by satisfaction. All kinds of results which various activities bring are termed as effect. It is quite easy to teach those activities which are learned by a feeling of pleasure or satisfaction. Students learn those activities in shortest time in which they feel pleasure while learning. Physical educator should have knowledge of this thing that which activities can be learnt by students with pleasure. Generally, students feel pleasure in learning those activities or sports in which they have interest. Physical educator should have knowledge of interest of all the students. While choosing the students for different sports, their interest should be taken into account.

Thus, processes of learning should be based on the rules or laws mentioned above. These rules state that if the students are not willing to participate in sports activities, they should be motivated by physical educator in such a way that they become attracted towards various physical activities. Students should be trained in such a way that they feel a kind of joy and also get feeling of satisfaction from learning. It is only with the help of this feeling that a physical educator can attain his goals, otherwise, his efforts will prove to be futile.

LAWS OF LEARNING

Edward L. Thorndike in the early 1900's postulated several "Laws of Learning," that seemed generally applicable to the learning process. Since that time, other educational psychologists have found that the learning process is indeed more complex than the "laws" identified. However, the "laws" do provide the instructor with insight into the learning process that will assist in providing a rewarding experience to the trainee.

The laws that follow are not necessarily stated as Professor Thorndike first stated them. Over the years, they have been restated and supplemented, but, in essence, they may be attributed to him. The first three are the basic laws: the law of readiness, the law of exercise, and the most famous and still generally accepted, the law of effect. The other three laws were added later as a result of experimental studies: the law of primacy, the law of intensity, and the law of recency.

As with anything else relative to the instruction and learning process, nothing that we do is a singular item; a combination of activities occurs at the same time to make the experience complete.

1. Law of Readiness

The Law of Readiness means a person can learn when physically and mentally adjusted (ready) to receive stimuli. Individuals learn best when they are ready to learn, and they will not learn much if they see no reason for learning. If trainees have a strong purpose, a clear objective and a sound reason for learning, they usually make more progress than trainees who lack motivation. When trainees are ready to learn, they are more willing to participate in the learning process, and this simplifies the instructor's job. If outside responsibilities or worries weigh heavily on trainees' minds or if their personal problems seem unsolvable, they may have little interest in learning.

2. Law of Exercise

The Law of Exercise stresses the idea that repetition is basic to the development of adequate responses; things most often repeated are easiest remembered. The mind can rarely recall new concepts or practices after a single exposure, but every time it is practiced, learning continues and is enforced. The instructor must provide opportunities for trainees to practice or repeat the task. Repetition consists of many types of activities, including recall, review, restatement, manual drill and physical application. Remember that practice makes permanent, not perfect unless the task is taught correctly.

3. Law of Effect

This law involves the emotional reaction of the learner. Learning will always be much more effective when a feeling of satisfaction, pleasantness, or reward accompanies or is a result of the learning process. Learning is strengthened when it is accompanied by a pleasant or satisfying feeling and that it is weakened when it is associated with an unpleasant experience. An experience that produces feelings of defeat, frustration, anger or confusion in a trainee is unpleasant. Instructors should be cautious about using negative motivation. Usually it is better to show trainees that a problem is not impossible, but is within their capability to understand and solve.

4. Law of Primacy

This law states that the state of being first, often creates a strong, almost unshakeable impression. For the instructor, this means that what they teach the first time must be correct. If a subject is incorrectly taught, it must be corrected. It is more difficult to un-teach a subject than to teach it correctly the first time. For the trainees' first learning experience should be positive and functionally related to training.

5. Law of Intensity

The principle of intensity states that if the stimulus (experience) is real, the more likely there is to be a change in behavior (learning). A vivid, dramatic or exciting learning experience teaches more than a routine or boring experience. A trainee will learn more from the real thing than from a substitute. Demonstrations, skits, and models do much to intensify the learning experiences of trainees.

6. Law of Recency

Things most recently learned are best remembered, while the things learned some time ago are remembered with more difficulty. It is sometimes easy, for example, to recall a telephone number dialed a few minutes ago, but it is usually impossible to recall a telephone number dialed a week ago. Review, warm-ups, and similar activities are all based on the principle that the more recent the exercise, the more effective the performance. Practicing a skill or new concept just before using it will ensure a more effective performance. Instructors recognize the law of recency when they plan a lesson summary or a conclusion of the lecture. Repeat, restate, or reemphasize important matters at the end of a lesson to make sure that trainees remember them instead of inconsequential details.

TRANSFER OF LEARNING

Transfer of training can be either positive or negative.

Positive transfer occurs when skills previously learned help, or facilitate the learning of a new skill. Negative transfer, on the other hand occurs when previous skill learning interferes with the learning of a new skill.

The direction of transfer in skill learning is said to depend upon the degree of response similarity in the previously learned and new tasks. The amount of positive or negative transfer is said to depend on the degree of stimulus similarity between the old and new tasks. For instance, if the stimuli in the old and new tasks are highly similar but conflicting responses must be made, transfer will be strongly negative.

Finally, we shall very briefly consider the transfer effects in verbal learning. As in skill learning, these can be positive or negative. Positive transfer occurs when things one has studies before help in new learning; negative transfer occurs when previously learned materials make it harder to learn new things. Most of the transfer is positive. Educational curricula are arranged so that there is often some overlap from course to course.

The practical aspect of learning is intimately bound up with the problem of the effect of learning one task upon the later learning of more or less different tasks. Will the training in performance of a given task, the acquisition of specific information and skill, help in dealing with other topics? There is the classical concept of 'formal discipline". Plato has asserted in the Republic that the practice of dancing, geometry and philosophy, would enable an individual to deal wisely with all possible social, economic or other practical situations. Many educational authorities, in the first quarter of this century, used to believe that a study of different classical languages like Latin and Greek had a definite moral value in building up 'character' and improving personality. Experimental studies however have falsified these hopes. In one of the earliest large-scale studies with school-subjects, the transfer-effects were found to be generally quite low, except where the subjects were more or less similar in content or methods. Later workers using much improved techniques have arrived at similar discouraging conclusions. A convenient summary was given by Thorndike (1924) and later by Woodworth (1948). The similarity of matter or of method between the two subjects was believed to lead to the so-called 'transfer-effect'. So the situation was described as a "transfer of "identical elements" '. Judd has put the opposite point of view claiming generalization from experience forward. He lays greater emphasis upon methods and principles. Since the training in any task implies some skill in methods as well as some insight into principles, any transfer-effect due to the use of similar methods and principles, can be ascribed to identities of procedure. The use of the term 'element' is somewhat disturbing; so it would be more accurate to talk of 'identical components'. When we talk of 'elements there is a convenient reference to reactions and nerve-conations that may be common to two tasks. Such a description, however suffers from the defect of being atomistic. But when we use terms like 'insight' and 'principles', there is an implicit possibility of extension and generalization.

The benefit of transfer from training in one subject to another is not free from interference due to nearness in time - the phenomenon of retroactive inhibition. It is well known that we can learn enough of a couplet to repeat the same correctly after one hearing. But if we hear once a series of 4 or 5 couplets one after the other, then it is often difficult to correctly recall even one of them. It appears that the impressions of the first experience are disturbed by the fresh impressions; and the latter interfere with the consolidation of the former. It is remarkable that the interference through retroactive inhibition increases in direct proportion with the amount of similarity between the preceding and the succeeding tasks. Thus a positive transfer-effect can be noticed only if sufficient time is allowed for rest between the two tasks of learning.

6

PHYSICAL EDUCATION AS A PROFESSION

Today physical education has become an important subject for all children. Hence, to help every child—the handicapped, the gifted, the disadvantaged, and the average—develop to the fullest of his or her interests and abilities in physical education is our professional commitment. Our greatest challenges is to provide quality education for all children. Equality of opportunity in physical education is meaningless unless instruction is relevant and of the highest quality appropriate for each child's learning needs. The demand for quality programs for all children is increasing, not decreasing. Strong pressures are making schools responsible for thinking through what kind of instruction is appropriate for each child.

A well-informed and demanding public is determined to see more effective instruction—what did the child learn and what did it cost? Support for programs is increasingly based upon clearly demonstrated student achievement on what is taught in the program. Physical educators must respond with valid, educationally defensible instructional programs. These programs must demonstrate their effectiveness in meeting the diverse needs of all children as they progress toward achieving the desired learning outcomes.

Two concepts—individualized instruction and accountability have been discussed in this chapter in beginning. Both of these concepts characterize quality programming in physical education for all. Significant features of the provisions of Public Law 94-142, Education for All Handicapped Children, underline free, appropriate public education and have implications for quality programs and physical education. These provisions as well as ways to meet the challenge for quality programming in physical education are presented.

Quality Programming: The Professional Imperative

Quality education always focus on the individual. Quality education is appropriate education for every child. Instruction, not students, must be adaptable to individual differences. Only in this way can we provide appropriate physical education for all students. The first step is a major one. It starts us on the course of increasing personalized instructional approaches to programming in physical education. Individualized instruction has long been singled out as a viable means of providing quality education for all children in that they are unique individuals who differ only in the nature of their learning needs.

Individual differences are described in terms that are directly relevant to instruction, not labels. Individualization requires us to stop typecasting the learner with labels such as special education, disadvantaged, poor gifted, or typically average. This approach has set us in pursuit of how to provide and deliver individualized instruction to meet every child's needs. Real individualization in physical education must begin with the acceptance of the learner as the central focus of concern.

In the past, the major focus of our concerns had been

fitting the student to the program, not the program to the student. Teaching in physical education school programs today does not often provide the opportunity for individualization such as:

i. assessing student's needs and abilities;

ii. setting student's learning tasks based on prior assessment data;

iii. prescribing and teaching based on assessment data;

iv. modifying instruction and learning tasks assigned based on student's achievement on objectives taught and covered in the lessons; and

v. involving students in planning, monitoring, and reporting results of instruction and parents in decision-making activities.

In this decade right to quality education for every student will become more pronounced. Strong pressures emerging as both national and state levels are calling for thorough and efficient education and equating these terms to quality education. Accountability has become one of the most easily identified features of quality education. In this sense, accountability is a key concept of this decade. It is relatively easy to focus on getting all children into some kind of physical education program designed to meet their needs. It is more difficult to ask whether or not this program works or how we measured its effectiveness—student's achievement of definitive goals of instruction. Individualization is observable in much of the accountability movement.

Accountability refers to the current trend in education to hold schools responsible for producing demonstrable learning in students on stated goals.

Accountability, when correctly implemented, can be an effective means for improving student learning, which is to provide impetus to discard what does not work and adopt new input approaches. Accountability is a tool, a systems-analysis approach to planning and evaluating instruction. It is focused on the desired student behaviours or "outputs" of the program. These "outputs" are cast in terms of observable and measurable results of instruction.

Evaluation of the effectiveness of the instructional program is based on these outputs—what did the student learn in the class? Measurements of "outputs", criterion-referenced levels of mastering objectives taught in the class, are being viewed as an effective strategy to improve schools. These measurements provide teachers with valuable feedback information that is critically needed in the process of individualizing instruction to meet the needs of the students in the class. Evaluating the effectiveness of the program in terms of student achievement will influence many decisions in state and local physical educational programs.

By demanding that we focus attention on the results of our programs, careful analysing and documenting is assured. We must know:

i. what our program goals are;

ii. what objectives should be achieved to reach these goals;

iii. what strategies we will use to plan and manage instruction for each learner to achieve desired outcomes;

iv. what our needs are to support quality programs.

In our society equity and quality education for all is

the value placed on each individual. In developing this rationale, we have increasingly emphasized the right of every child to quality programs—instructions appropriate to each child's learning needs. Physical education for a child who has special needs is not a charity. It is not a desired extra in school programs. It is a fundamental right to which a child and the child's family are entitled. Although the following section deals specifically with legal and policy mandates that require greater imperative is to develop quality programs, individualized and accountable, for all children as we step toward the twenty-first century.

Teaching-Learning: Task-Oriented, Orderly, Motivating, Safe

For teaching and learning there should be a task-oriented and free of threat of failure on assigned learning task climate. Main purpose of teaching-learning climate is to organize the class in such a manner by which available time can be fully utilised. All teaching and learning activities reflect a sense of purposefulness.

Students and teachers know the objectives of instruction. The lesson is organized to maximize instructional time for learning assigned tasks. High-interest activities are provided to engage students in learning assigned tasks. The learning tasks assigned are challenging—not too difficult nor too easy—providing a high degree of success for all students. The setting is relatively clean, safe from physical threat or harm, and accessible to all students.

Students know what is expected of them and the imposition of discipline is uniform for all. Help is provided to students with learning difficulties. Teachers supply feedback-reinforcement as soon as possible.

Student progress is monitored continuously and instructional activities are adapted accordingly. Students are presented directives by teachers. Drill, practice and organized game-time activities are provided to the whole class group and assigned as independent learning contracts according to students' abilities. Students are actively involved in planning, coaching skills, reporting results, and helping each other for at least 60% of the instructional time.

Monitoring Student Progress and Using Measures of Student Achievement as the Basis for Program Evaluation

Student progress is measured and reported frequently. The results of assessments are used to improve individual student performance and to improve the instructional program. The feedback from assessment of student performance is a valuable source of information for teachers when teachers believe that student achievement is derived largely from instruction. The teachers use student achievement data as the basis of program effectiveness: whether or not to continue the program or teaching-learning activity.

Teachers are willing to accept the fact that the best way to evaluate student progress is to collect measures of pupil performance frequently. The measures of performance do not rely on teacher judgment alone or on teacher judgment in combination with grades assigned for a unit of activity. Although useful, such measures do not provide adequate curriculum-based assessments of skill mastery. Multiple measures need to be used, which should reinforce one another. Criterion-referenced measurements are preferred to norm-referenced measurements.

A norm-referenced measurement is a standardized achievement test. This measurement communicates little about the student's actual skills and performance levels on what is taught in the class. It answers the questions: "How much has Tom improved since last year" and "Is his achievement at, above, or below that of a representative sampling of students his age, grade, sex, state or region?" The criterion measures permit teachers to individually analyse each student's progress. Students are not evaluated in comparison with each other. They are evaluated in comparison to the uniform standard of mastery to which all students are expected to rise. Criterion-referenced evaluation procedures can be used by teachers in four different types of testing programs.

First, criterion-referenced tests are used for pre-assessment of students on objectives taught in instruction. Second, criterioning the progress of students so teachers can help students who are having difficulties when necessary. Third, they are used to modify components of instruction for student objectives and instructional procedures. Fourth, criterion-referenced tests are used at the end of the instructional unit, grade or program level to determine whether students have achieved the criterion levels of objectives taught. It is recommended that criterion-referenced measures be locally validated, curriculum-based standardized measures.

These measures ensure that students are tested on what they are taught. The measure is validated to be certain that the description of mastery is an acceptable level of mastery for all students in the school program. The measure is standardized so as to eliminate teacher subjectivity as a possible source of error or unfairness in assessing student progress.

Parent Involvement and Other Citizen in the Educational System

Positive experiences with active parent involvement in education resulted in communities establishing broader of education coalitions. These coalitions become more deeply involved in broader educational processes and develop positive feelings and support for school program goals and objectives. To improve quality education, effective schools deem it essential to strive to foster mutual school-community relations.

Every effort is made to actively involve parents and other citizens in the educational processes: planning the program, implementing the program, evaluating the effectiveness of the program, and communicating results of the program to the community-at-large. Parents and other citizens can be involved as:

1. Decision Advisors. Many federal and state guidelines recommend or require parental involvement in programs receiving federal or state funds. Because of this requirement, more parents have become involved in assisting with decision-making. Encouraging parents in this role brings about shared responsibility for decisions and the change to quality decisions is increased.

2. Educational Monitors. Parents are informed through regular communication procedures of happenings in the school district or of a particular program. They are encouraged to attend board of education meetings, advisory meetings, and to participate as members of planning committees.

3. Community Organizers. Many parents and other citizens excel in organizational skills for a common

purpose. These individuals can reach people in many organizations and other agencies, inform them of issues related to quality education, or recruit others to help to improve the school program. They can link the school programs with resource people in the community who can assist teachers in enriching through presentations or availability of community resources.

Instructional Leadership and Support Services

The mission of the school and the individual programs within the school can be effectively communicate to the staff, parents, students and community-at-large by instructional leaders. The leader understands and applies the characteristics of instructional effectiveness in the management of the instructional program. The leader ensures open communication and organized support services for all involved in schooling. Accepting the premise that the instructional program is directed toward accomplishing specific goals and objectives, then it follows that teachers and the school-community-at-large expect certain leadership qualities and behaviours from the principal: goal-setting, assessment and accountability, support, information, supervision and building a working consensus of quality programs for all students. Communication focuses on the "what" and "why" of instructional programs, effective practices, assessing school and teaching effectiveness and determining in-service education needs to improve competence and productivity.

The principal of the school or facility provides organized support services and effective delivery of these services to both teachers and students. Effective school programs depend on the acceptance and cooperation among teachers, administrators, parents, and students as well as the availability and allocation of physical resources and equipment. The design of strategies for delivering these needed supports to teachers is a major leadership task in implementing effective program.

Teachers may require training in effective use of available support services to maximize their effectiveness in meeting the needs of all students. Teachers are challenged to become broadly resourceful in maintaining more flexible and diverse learning environments, seeking and collaborating with others who have expertise in meeting special needs. If the instructional program is to be effective, leadership must be provided and consideration must be given to specifying the kind and extent of supportive services that are needed to best serve the teachers and all the students in the regular class.

Criteria for Designing a Model for Quality Programming

Definition of quality programs, effective practices, and benefits for all participants involved in the educational process are criteria for designing quality programs. The participants include students, teachers, parents, administrators, boards of education, legislators, and other members of the school community. Six major criteria were derived for designing quality programs. These criteria are analogous to categories.

Within each category there are specific statements of specifications. Some of these specifications have been identified for each criterion. These criteria are following:

i. Flexibility

1. Clearly defined program goals, common to all students, with a wide range of content exemplified by objectives to meet unique needs of individual students,

districts, schools and/or classrooms.

2. Objectives pursued within a given class group are readily adaptable to meet unique needs of learners at all levels.

3. Instructional activity options to meet the unique needs of learners within a given class are readily available to all student at all levels.

ii. Accountability

1. The program provides for systematic monitoring of student progress and frequent reporting of student achievement results to all members of the school community.

2. The program provides systematic procedures for using the results of instruction (student achievement on stated learning outcomes), to improve individual student performance as well as the program.

3. The program provides for criterion levels of objectives to help teachers individually analyse each student's progress on a uniform standard of mastery to which all students are expected to rise.

iii. Communication

1. The program's mission, instructional focus and direction, is clearly articulated and readily communicated to students, parents, administrators, colleagues and other relevant members of the school community.

2. A program plan, documented program goals and relevant essential objectives by grade or multi-levels to achieve these goals, serves as a communication tool for establishing common agreement and understanding between teachers, students, parents and administrators.

3. The program plan serves as a communicating tool for students to understand self-confidence. All students are expected to learn essential skills.

4. The program plan provides a structure for parent involvement, namely, by understanding the specific instructional requirements and student expectancies, resources needed to support the program, and reinforcing goals of the program.

5. The program structure clearly defines the teaching competency requirements to effectively implement instruction for all students alike.

iv. Compliance

1. The program must provide for full compliance with state and federal legal mandates and policies, and professional guideline standards.

2. The program affords a structure to facilitate continuous updating of instructional processes with new educational and technological research and development practices.

v. Efficiency

1. The program goals and objectives serve to organize and provide sequential, progressive non-redundant program content maximizing the available instructional time and resources—equipment, materials and support services for teachers and students.

2. The program provides a student data base on clearly defined objectives to help teachers plan, implement and evaluate the effectiveness of their instruction—student achievement.

3. The program provides a consistent framework to yield data—units of improvement—to properly document

programmatic needs—improve quality and/or defend the program.

vii. Effectiveness

1. The teachers must demonstrate the stated level of mastery of the teaching behaviours required to implement the program as intended.

2. The program must result in a significant number of student (high proportion) demonstrating mastery on the essential skills specified for instruction.

Using these criteria to select, select/adapt, or design a quality program, a curriculum model that invariably emerges is based on objectives for instruction and evaluation.

TRAINING COURSE

1. 2 years certificate course for 10+2 (C.P.Ed.)

2. For 10+2 qualified:- 3 years degree courses (B.P.Ed.)

3. For Graduates - One year diploma course (D.P.Ed.)

4. For Graduates - One year degree course (B.P.Ed.)

5. One year graduate course having physical education as a compulsory subject.

6. Two years post-graduate physical education course (M.P.Ed.)

7. One year Post-graduate Education Course.

8. Post-graduate (Arts) (Physical Education) and Post-graduate Science (Physical Education) Two Year course

PHYSICAL EDUCATION IS NOW A VIABLE CAREER OPTION

Looking for a career in sports and physical education? If you are, there is now no need to be disheartened.

Academics from some of India's prominent universities running these courses say there are opportunities galore in the field, since health is a cause for increasing concern among the teeming millions of India.

Universities and other educational institutions have also realised the importance of sports and physical education as a viable career option as well. "Health has always been a matter of great concern for us. But now in this fast moving world we are neglecting it as we don't have time for ourselves," said V Satyanarayana, head of the department of physical education in Osmania University, Hyderabad.

"This is the place where the need for a specialist physical instructor comes in. Nowadays, we have become health conscious and are joining gyms, yoga and aerobics classes and specialists in these fields are much in demand," he said. Osmania University, which produced cricketers like ML Jaisimha and Mohammed Azharuddin, as well as, renowned sports broadcaster Harsha Bhogle, offers physical education courses in both under-graduate and post-graduate levels.

Similar courses are also available in Guru Nanak Dev University, Amritsar, and Lakshmibai National Institute of Physical Education (LNIPE), Gwalior, which is the only deemed university in Asia in the field. Calcutta, Bangalore and Kerala universities also have such degree and postgraduate courses.

Not to be left behind, Delhi University has now decided to start a three-year degree course from the current academic year. It also plans to start a master's course well before the first batch graduates. Over half a dozen colleges affiliated to the university have already agreed to introduce the course and admissions are expected to start soon.

"There is increasing interest in sports in our country. And there is a need for proper training and guidance to these enthusiasts. So we are promoting physical education and sports science as a subject in various universities," University Grants Commission chairman SK Thorat said.

The physical education course is divided in two parts – theory and application. The former deals with the science of physical education while the latter involves practical training in different sporting activities, fitness programmes, aerobics, gym operations, sports and event management and also sports journalism. LNIPE Vice-Chancellor Shibnath Mukhrejee feels this is a wide field and students opting for specialised courses in physical education and sports sciences can also get into coaching and psychology and team management.

"There has been an urgent need to redefine the concepts of physical education and coaching in different sports. Coaches need to stay up-to-date in order to face the challenges posed by sports academies and coaching centres," he said.

"Students who opt for such courses land up with coaching and other sports related jobs. We also have certificate programmes for coaches and only persons who have represented at least their university in a sport are eligible." Mukherjee added that LNIPE, run by the ministry of sports and youth affairs, also offers an adventure sports course which help people gain international assignments, thanks to the booming tourism sector.

7

LEADERSHIP

MEANING OF LEADER

A person who directs and co-ordinates activities of an organised group, which attempt to achieve specific goal or goals, is known as Leader. All the functions performed by leaders with the aim of motivating or guiding the players is known as leadership. Only that leader can prove to be effective, who influence the behaviour of group members to considerable extent. A leader who is unable to alter the behaviours and attitudes of group members cannot be considered as an effective leader.

Today's competitive world, where all the players participate with the aim of winning the championship, role of leaders has increased tremendously. This is the main reason that concept of leadership and functions performed by leaders are being discussed in length in this chapter. A coach can make a difference in the player's sport performance and team success, leadership skills count in performance of team and players. All the players who participate in competitions are human beings and not machine, because of which they get affected to a lot of extent by attitudes, behaviours and personality of leader. Main responsibility which lies on shoulder of team leader is to help each competitor to reach his or her true potential. For this, it is very important that coach must know about his functions and importance. In field of sports, generally name of Coach is provided to leader, who mould the behaviours and attitudes of players to considerable extent.

Roles in which a Coach Functions

It is not an easy task to influence and mould the behaviours of players and to fill them with required self-confidence for competition. Players are human beings because of which they differ from each other as to type of personal approach with which they are most comfortable. All coaches are not able to meet individual needs of the players.

Actually, the best coaches are secure individuals. They recognise their strengths and limitations and they do not get satisfied with their level of knowledge. To make continuous development in level of knowledge, they attend various seminars and take help of professional literature for this purpose. They also consult with specialists and professionals to change a particular approach. For this reason, it is very necessary for the coaches to possess some personal and technical skill. To meet each of these skills, it becomes necessary for the leaders or coaches to maintain a variety of roles, some of which can be explained in following manner:—

a. Leader : When more than one person attempts to attain a specific goal, it becomes necessary to provide their efforts a proper direction to appoint someone as their in charge or leader. In sports activities, role of in charge is performed by coach. All the players assume that their coach will provide a sense of leadership to achieve group success. For providing such kind of feeling, it is necessary for him to direct them towards a specific goal. For effective leadership, it becomes necessary for the coach to assume some responsibilities on his shoulders. For instance, for making all arrangements during training and for preparing post-game strategies. If a leader take responsibility of team failure on him, then players will feel sense of leadership to a lot of extent.

b. Teacher : Coaches are not different from teachers. In reality, effective coaches are educators. Players who make progress in developing their skills become more creative, self-assured and successful. Educational process in sports is to teach players to think independently of directions provided by coach and to respond creatively to unanticipated actions of their opponents.

Only those coaches prove to be effective, who have thorough knowledge of skills and strategies used in the sport. Likewise, it is very important to have an ability to communicate this knowledge to others. It is very important for the coaches to have ability to communicate their knowledge to their players so that they can applied it appropriately in competitions. Best coaches make use of various means to upgrade their skills and knowledge.

To become an effective teacher, it is necessary for the coach to ask his players about the effectiveness of his or her teaching. He should keep on changing the modes of communication from time to time, as continuous use of same technique can arise feeling of boreness in them. Coach should provide specific kind of feedback to players which they can use in a relatively non-hostile way. Coach should not provide knowledge of new skills during the contest, but rehears them in practice until participants can perform them comfortably and properly.

c. Follower : Coaches should be follower of players not in the sense that should make design programmes and strategies in accordance with need and wishes of players, but in the sense that should provide them respect and dignity whenever required. A good coach knows when not to lead the players and when to respect the decisions taken by players. One should not consider strategy of following as a weakness, rather it can prove to be a strength if applied appropriately. The group leader should not constantly demonstrate dominance. Coach can prove to be more effective by allowing captains and other players of the team responsible for certain team related tasks. Such kind of freedom and opportunities fill the players with a sense of dignity and self-respect, with which they get motivated to work harder.

d. Limit Setter : Only that coach can prove to be effective, who can analyse realistic capacities of the players. Various kinds of demands are put on players, some of which include: maintenance of proper training and conforming to team policies. Sometimes, it becomes necessary for the coach to restrict and set limits on certain behaviours so that players can be prepare properly for outstanding performance in competition.

It is necessary to develop and implement the guidelines and specific procedures for monitoring the player's adherence. As the limit setter, various choices or alternatives remain available with coach. He can modify the rules, can ask for more player input and even can explain various matters among players which are not negotiable. Sometimes it becomes necessary and desirable for the coaches to set limit, as it provides help to him in controlling certain actions of players. Peer pressure to test rules and to go along with the gang becomes overwhelming. For this reason, this role should be performed by coach very carefully.

d. Role Model : No learning process can take place without setting any standard or example to which learner's can imitate or by which their ability can be compared. Such kind of standard or example is called Model. In demonstration proper or sportsmanlike behaviour, coaches serve as models for their players. Coaches must be consistence in following the similar rules and expectations in their own actions and attitudes that they expect of their players.

No coach can expect his players to avoid those bad habits, which are found in himself. By working with double standards, he cannot get satisfactory and proper results. In reality, to maintain a double standard in regard to team policies is to invite distrust and a loss of credibility. No coach can inspire the players to keep themselves neat and clean unless he does not keep himself neat. Thus, only that coach can be consider a successful one, who can set himself as a role model in front of players.

e. Friend : Coaches should relate themselves with players in such a way as they are in same peer group and have interests of their players. However, this should be done to a limited extent, because it is very necessary that players should admire and respect their coaches. The attitude towards coaches and friends should be different. In reality, player's expectations of coach's behaviours and attitudes differ from those of their friends. If coach will try to become or behave with players like their friends to lot of extent, then players themselves will tend to feel uncomfortable.

No doubt that an element of friendship should exist in healthy relationship existing between player and coach, but extent of this should be controllable. Coaches should be available to interact in a meaningful way with every player, even away from the sport arena. Coaches can get players out of trouble, lend them money, pat them on the back, laugh, cry and cheer with them, and not let anyone else talk about them. Thus, a relationship built on trust, honesty, disclosure of feelings to a degree, can be a healthy friendship, but this should not be done to such an extent, that players do not respect their coaches, considering him as to be their friend.

f. Substitute of Parent : It is very necessary for the stable children to have someone around them who cares about them and who is important in their life. One must have the love and concern of a significant other, someone who really matters. The role of coach is not to become parent of player, but to support the same goals that parents have for their player children. As the role model for players, coach has to carried out a host of parental functions.

Role as parent gets magnified when the athlete has a single parent. No coach should make use of abusive language, embarrassing and insulting comments. It is necessary that between coach and players, an agreement about future behaviours should be conducted, as without this, relationship of trust and respect cannot be developed among them.

g. Counsellor : For performing function of coaching properly, it is not necessary for the coach to be rude and over strict with players. In reality, effective coaches are not threatening to their players, and the players in turn feel that they can risk communicating most thoughts to the coach. In this kind of atmosphere, the coach can listen and respond to needs and requirements of each player, which is important if the coach wants players to perform without thoughts and feelings that interfere with performance preparation and participation.

It is desirable to have airing out of feelings inhibiting full concentration to the task. In the beginning of career, especially various kinds of negative thinking and fear gets aroused in players. Coach should listen to them carefully and try to help players in overcoming them. Not only this, if players have any kind of problem, he should pay attention to them also and try to sort out that problem in such a way that player's performance cannot get affected in any way.

Thus from above discussion it can be said that there are various roles in which a coach has to function and only that coach can be consider a successful one, which can perform all the functions in above mentioned roles properly.

To understand the concept and nature of leadership and to determine the manner in which function of leadership can be performed effectively, various theories have been designed by experts. Effective leadership behaviour is impossible to dictate for all situations and players. Scholars who examine the interactions between a group leader and the group's member are unable to prescribe any single best leadership approach. This is particular true in sports activities, where participants who differ in various respect from each other. It has been found that it is necessary to make use of different kinds of approaches in different sports activities. It is very difficult to predict success based on certain leadership characteristics. Even the definition and meaning of success gets differ in various sports activities. From various leadership theories, some recommendations have been derived, which can be described in following manner :—

a. While making or designing plans and programs for the players, it is necessary for the coaches to take into account the feelings and abilities of players. It can be said that effective managers of groups should be tune in to requirements of members of team. Member of all groups tend to feel greater satisfaction with group goals if they have played a part in creating and carrying out these goals, alongwith the rules and expected behaviours. It is not necessary for the players to create and implement all the rules themselves, but they can have their own individual feelings and requirements, which a coach take into account.

b. Different kinds of techniques prove to be successful in different sports activities. This can be mention in the way that there cannot be any best way to lead for all situations. Coaches in golf and basketball differ markedly as to the leadership style that best fosters athletic performance. It becomes necessary for the coaches to make critical assessment of their unique situations and surroundings before making use of any training technique.

c. It is necessary for the coach to motivate the players to perform outstandingly in competitions. Competent coaches try to develop various kinds of qualities in players, but it does not happen on its own. A coach cannot simply command and expect to receive respect, loyalty and credity. The liked and respected leader does not need formal power.

Actually, leadership is not built on intimidation, fear and completion of tasks, rather effective leaders earn the respect of their subordinates through honesty, mutual respect, empathy and sincerity and the ability to teach skills efficiently.

d. In all sports activities, different kinds of skills are used, without which no one can become outstanding player of that sport. Very few players or learners come to the sport arena with the necessary sport skills and proper attitude and mental training to compete successfully. The task of giving them knowledge about skills of game and also to provide proper direction to attitude of children or player rest with coach. In reality, an effective coach teaches mental and physical skills or at least provide skill learning situations to players. To ensure that each player has grow and has become maturer, he take necessary time and exert the required energy.

e. There should be a balance between task and relationship oriented styles. Efficiency of that team will remain lower whose member do not like each other. Member satisfaction through affiliation helps teammates to support one another. Receiving recognition, respect and support from teammates is an important need for most players. It is not mutually exclusive to complete tasks to reach goals and to maintain healthy relationships among group members. This applies more to young players who have a greater need to establish meaningful relationships with their coach as compared to experienced and higher skilled players.

The manner in which a coach is being perceived by group or team members is determined to a lot of extent by the style or technique that he uses for his purpose. Group's perception of leader is more important than effectiveness of leader's behaviour. Often in sports activities, player's perception of their coach dictates loyalty and respect. Thus, it can be said that technique which a coach uses defines the effectiveness of his function to a lot of extent.

Concept of Successful and Effective Leadership

The ability to get others to behave as the manager intends them to behave is being termed as successful leadership. Even after satisfaction of coach's needs, it is possible that player's needs remain ignored. Generally, it is found that coaches give attention to young or inexperienced players, while ignore altogether to experienced ones. In case of effective leadership, players perform according to coach's intentions and desires and at the same time satisfy their own needs.

Thus, it can be said that success has to do only with getting the job done, while effectiveness adds the concept of satisfaction on the part of those who do the job. In this manner, positive feelings of subordinates usually contribute to long-term benefits such as team loyalty, support and enjoyment of participation, which is an important component of intrinsic motivation. Resolving conflicts in absence of teammates certainly contribute to team and coach loyalty. Thus, effective coaches are concerned with maintaining good relationships with team members for a long period of time.